# YOGA

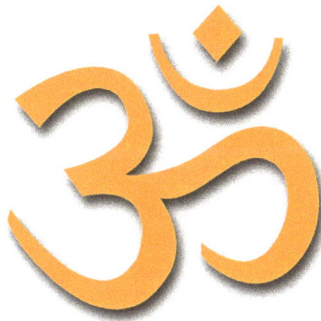

## KEEPING IT UP

PAMELA MARIKO

FORDHAM PUBLISHING AUSTRALIA

NOTE: This book portrays general stretches, warm-ups, yoga drawn from
different traditions and yoga breathing exercises. It includes guidance
for meditation, stress management, relaxation and diet for wellbeing.

# Dedication

*To my students and all who strive for
health and peace on all levels of being.*

# CONTENTS

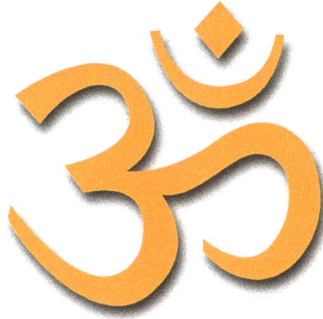

## INTRODUCTION

This book is not intended to be an in-depth or academic text on yoga, but rather to assist to in the practice of basic yoga when the student is unable to attend a class. Firstly, here is a very brief introduction to a much deeper subject:

Yoga is about creating balance within the body, mind and emotions so that we can live in peace, good health and harmony with the greater whole. Around 200 AD the foundations of yoga philosophy were written in *The Yoga Sutra of Patanjali*. It describes the inner workings of the mind and provides an eight-step template for mastering a restless mind and harnessing peace.

# THE EIGHT LIMBS OF YOGA

| | |
|---|---|
| **YAMA**<br>**Universal morality** | Ethical restraints: Ahimsa: Non-violence, harmlessness in thought, word, deed to people, creatures, self and things. Satya: Non-lying. Others: Non-stealing. Sense control. Non-greed. Non-attachment; moderation. |
| **NIYAMA**<br>**Personal observances** | Purity, cleanliness. Modesty; contentment. Discipline; effort. Self-study/examination/reflection. Cultivation of peace. Awareness of Divinity as a guiding force. Making time to connect with God/the Divine. |
| **ASANA**<br>**Body postures** | Postural exercises that help the individual to explore and control concentration. Postures act as a link between the physical, emotional and ethereal bodies. |
| **PRANAYAMA**<br>**Breath control** | Breathing exercises beneficial to mind and body. The measuring, control and directing of breath balances the body's vital forces. Pranayama strengthens the respiratory system, soothes nerves and reduces craving. |
| **PRATYHARA**<br>**Sense withdrawal** | Drawing back; retreating from that which stimulates the senses. |
| **DHARANA**<br>**Concentration** | Concentration of the mind. To focus on one object or point until mind, intellect and ego are restrained. |
| **DHYANA**<br>**Meditation** | Meditation on the Divine. Devotion. The mind is still and quiet, leading to a subconscious function. |
| **SAMADHI** | Oneness with universal energy. Bliss. Nirvana. |

Imagine this as a pyramid, with the building blocks at the bottom of the structure being YAMA, to include: truthfulness, non-stealing; sense control, non-greed, non-attachment; moderation and non-violence in thought, word and deed.

Thoughts are living things. Yoga teaches that there are three states created by our thoughts: creation, preservation and destruction. Whether peaceful, positive, angry or negative, these thoughts are in the energy field around us and can travel through time and space. They are picked up by others and create our reality.

You can't 'un-say' something, so we must choose our words carefully.

Deeds: The quality of harmlessness should extend towards all Beings from the smallest flying or crawling type, to humanity and larger mammals, birds and fish.

It begins at home, in the workplace and within social and community groups as practice for extending beyond. You might think of wars, crimes against humanity, live export, animal experimentation, intensive farming, puppy and kitten farms, skin trade and how skins are taken from animals in some countries, and so on. Non-violence is reflected in the yoga diet which is vegetarian, and for many, vegan.

The second step up is NIYAMA, self-observances; self-study. In the western world and in a secular sense, this can be likened to study of psychology: the psychology of observing the self, such as a moral review, a character review and studying reactions and thought patterns. Mystery schools of east and west have long propagated the study of self to become aware of thought processes and behaviour. Observing and practising these philosophies will assist in the journey of self.

Hatha yoga: your body is your temple. It houses the soul force. It is your responsibility to keep it in good working order.

Your body is animated by prana, which is much more than just breath. It is life force, soul. After all, the first breath animates the body with a living force. When the last breath is taken, the physical body is no longer animated by that 'force'. So, it is important to fill the lungs with this magical source of life, preferably outside or near an open window. Pranayama is to measure and control prana with breathing exercises.

If you can withdraw the senses, you can be still, in a space in your mind slightly removed from everyday reality. This is good preparation for concentration.

Concentration trains the mind to focus, narrowing the field of focus to one-pointedness in preparation for meditation.

Meditation may be experienced differently by individuals. The dictionary definition states: A reverential act of entering complete conceptual and intellectual silence (not daydreaming). Initially you may be aware of your thoughts, without interacting with them: being master of them - rather than your thoughts being master of you. With practice, meditation can be like waves of consciousness, too vague to be considered thoughts, but more of a blending with a higher reality.

This can lead your consciousness to blend back into the universe for seconds, minutes, or perhaps longer. This oneness is known as samadhi - oneness with universal energy. It is the aim of meditation to lead to samadhi.

Yoga is not a religion. It means unity. Unity with a higher force. This force is perceived by individuals in many ways. It can mean connection with whatever your perception of a higher reality is. This may be connecting to your higher self, your inner self, Divine reality, the Cosmic, God, Jehovah, Allah, Buddha, The Goddess, Mother Earth, outer space, the 'God of your heart' whatever you conceive him, her, it or them to be - or as George Lucas, the creator of Star Wars so succinctly puts it, 'The Force'.

See the pyramid on the following page.

**THE EIGHT LIMBS OF YOGA**

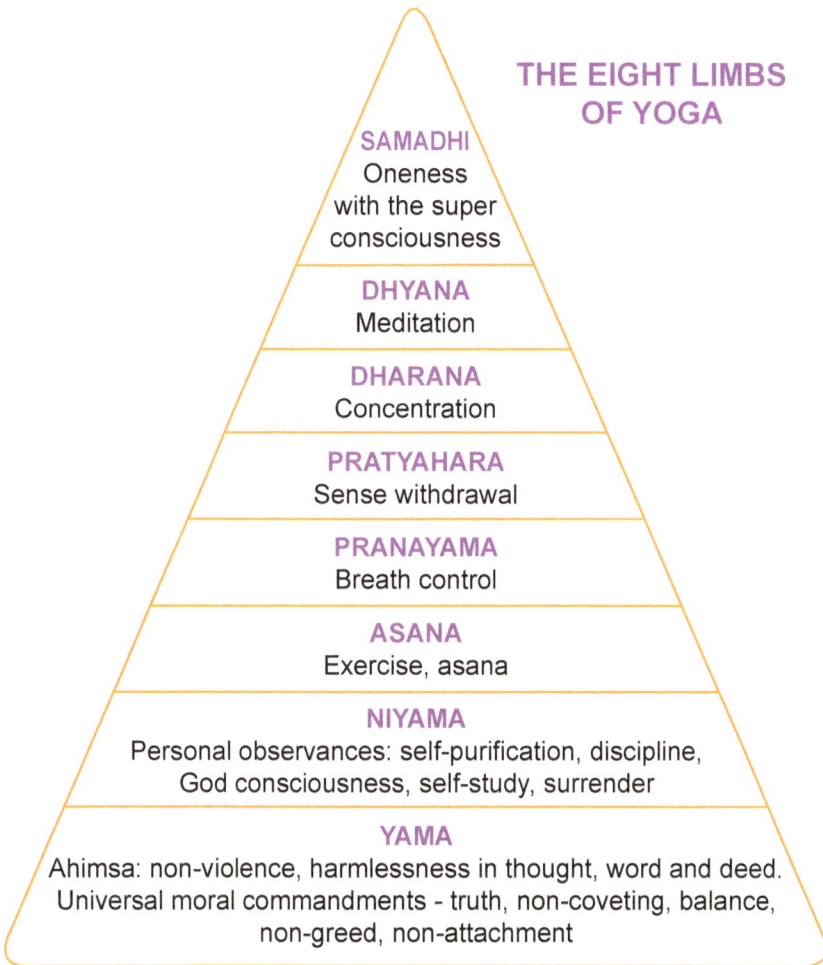

**SAMADHI**
Oneness with the super consciousness

**DHYANA**
Meditation

**DHARANA**
Concentration

**PRATYAHARA**
Sense withdrawal

**PRANAYAMA**
Breath control

**ASANA**
Exercise, asana

**NIYAMA**
Personal observances: self-purification, discipline, God consciousness, self-study, surrender

**YAMA**
Ahimsa: non-violence, harmlessness in thought, word and deed. Universal moral commandments - truth, non-coveting, balance, non-greed, non-attachment

Let's assume you are kind to all living Beings or thinking about being so; are conscious of what you are eating and are considering your dietary choices. You're keen to improve the body. Additionally, you are working on the self, psychologically speaking: mindful of thoughts and actions.

Being mindful is an ancient Buddhist and Hindu concept of being present and aware all the time: each step you take, each action you perform and each word you utter.

If you are keen to focus the mind, stabilise the emotions; minimise stress and experience peace and harmony in life, how, you might ask, will yoga postures help?

## THE BENEFITS OF YOGA

Hatha Yoga exercise improves flexibility and strength, but more importantly works on the autonomic nervous system and the endocrine glands to keep the body healthy.

Long before medical science knew anything about the endocrine glands, people in India were practising asanas (postures) to regulate the function of these glands.

The endocrine glands have influence on the emotions and nervous system. They are governors of our lives and affect how we react to situations. You could say that they are like psychic receptors.

When performing yoga asanas, some of the glands receive a massage and tone. By stimulating these organs and glands, together with correct breathing and relaxation techniques, the practice helps balance the emotions, calm the mind; aid a positive outlook and build confidence.

Additionally, we are preparing the body at a base level, to be receptive, and 'in tune', heightening our awareness.

This is explained more fully under the heading of 'STRESS', in Section 9.

In summary, yoga postures work on the inner body and its subtle faculties - as well as the outer muscles.

There are specific postures for conditions such as asthma, backache, lack of libido and just about any other ailment you can think of.

When we exercise, we release hormones called endorphins, and these endorphins make us feel good and become more optimistic about life. You know how it is - when you feel good and positive you attract things into your life. People respond to you more positively, generally, and more good things happen.

We also release these and other hormones when we laugh. If, however, you don't exercise, you aren't releasing endorphins like the person who is exercising daily, unless you are rolling about laughing all day.

Endorphins - they are worth exercising for.

You don't have to be double jointed or super flexible to do yoga. It is not a competition. It is a case of yoga being good to you, not 'how good you are' at it. Besides, practice makes perfect - or at least - better.

I started yoga in my mid-twenties - several decades ago. I had never been sporty, nor was I a ballerina. In fact, when I was a teenager, it was trendy to slump, with long hair forward, face hanging between rounded shoulders.

As for breathing: I enjoyed the odd cigarette in the bicycle sheds during the last year at school, rather than hockey (but have since corrected both my shoulders and the error of my ways).

This book portrays some stretches, warm-ups, basic hatha yoga postures and easy variations for some of them. Hatha is the umbrella term which covers all yoga postures (asanas) otherwise known as yoga exercise.

## HATHA YOGA

There are umpteen different yoga styles these days: traditional classical yoga, such as Iyengar yoga, developed by BKS Iyengar; Ashtanga formulated by Pattabhi Jois, Vinyasa - of the Ashtanga strain, and the yoga taught by Satyananda and Sivananda yoga schools, to name but a few. Swami Satyananda was a disciple of Sivananda. The two styles are similar and include meditation and chanting. Both styles are gentler than those mentioned above.

Imagine these names like Smith Yoga, Brown Yoga, Jones Yoga, Harding Yoga and so-on. Whatever 'strain' it is, if referring to exercise, it comes under the banner of HATHA yoga, meaning effort, force or exertion.

You may have heard that HA is known to be symbolic of the sun, SURYA, and THA the moon, CHANDRA. HA and THA don't mean 'sun' and 'moon' but they provide an analogy about the two sides of ourselves.

For example, there are left and right nerve channels in the subtle body called NADIS which are associated with lunar and solar forces: IDA the left, and PINGALA the right, being the left and right nostrils, left and right sides of the spine and of the body. These carry life force energies and the flow of consciousness, or prana, in the physical and subtle bodies.

We'll use the word subtle body throughout to indicate the non-physical. You can equate the subtle body to 'psychic body' which includes layers of everything that we are. Some call it astral body, yet that is only one small part of what it is.

The two NADIS are believed to be stimulated through different breathing practices including NADI SHODHANA, alternate nostril breathing, explained towards the end of the book. This stimulates the left and right sides of the brain respectively.

The NADIS correspond to moon and sun, female and male, anima and animus, yin and yang, cold and hot, passive and active. They are composed of negatively and positively charged ions. You could equate them to the duality we are in every way: our physical and our subtle bodies, our light and dark sides, and so on.

Breathing through the left, the lunar energy or passive side, stimulates the right side of the brain - the creative, more dreamy side. Breathing through the right, solar energy or active side, stimulates the left brain: the analytical, logical side.

Since hatha means exertion or force, it could be argued that by working with the force and the breath, we strive to bring the pillars of opposites within ourselves into better balance - even though there will always be fluctuation.

Just as there are a multitude of physical asanas and

pranayama exercises, there are also many different types of yoga.

We have already covered that HATHA YOGA is the umbrella term for yoga involving the body by performing ASANAS, and PRANAYAMA YOGA is about exercises involving the restraint or control of the breath, which is the life force.

Here are a few of the other types of yoga:

BHAKTI YOGA is the yoga of love and devotion or worship. It can be the love of others or humanity in general.

KARMA YOGA is work, service or selfless action.

JNANA YOGA is the yoga of sacred knowledge; the meditation on higher truths/the self.

These embody aspects of YAMA and NIYAMA - the building blocks of yoga.

There is now a wave of new yoga over the last two decades, somewhat removed from the early teachings of 'working on the self' including the ego, in order to be in tune with the universe, or more succinctly - closer to God.

On the plus side, it could be contended that the more modern gym-type yoga classes could be a platform to a deeper study of yoga.

The yoga in this book is mainly sourced from the more traditional/classical yoga strains and only touches on the deeper aspects. Unless you are doing only meditation, which is RAJA yoga, most students are doing hatha yoga, with some pranayama (breathing exercises) and maybe some meditation at the end of the class (raja yoga) and relaxation. Some types of yoga relaxation are known as YOGA NIDRA - which means psychic sleep. The subconscious becomes active and the conscious mind rests. The subconscious merges with the unconscious.

Slow yogic breathing known as pranayama, is part and parcel of yoga practice. In the latter part of this book we'll address some common pranayama exercises. As you perform yoga asanas, take your awareness into each breath and each movement, extending, not over-stretching. Maintain the posture for a few breaths or a few seconds as is comfortable.

## A Word of Warning

If you have any concerns about your back, neck or other body part, or are pregnant, **please check with a medical professional** before commencing yoga.

If you have had a slipped disc or burst disc, then spinal twists and some stronger back stretches will *not* be appropriate.

During pregnancy, some postures are helpful, others not recommended.

Females shouldn't do shoulder-stands, half shoulder-stands or headstands during the days of menstruation.

High or low blood pressure and or propensity to feeling faint, needs careful management.

Having said this, I have had a wonderful 82 year-young lady in my classes, several in their seventies, young pregnant women, students with stents, lupus, fibromyalgia, scoliosis and dowager's humps. I have taught builders with spinal and back issues and the bionic brigade with metal hips, knees, back parts and so on. All have enjoyed improved health and mobility, but both student and teacher need to be aware and modify poses.

When attending classes, always let a yoga teacher know of any medical condition, muscle, ligament or bone challenge, stitches, or pregnancy.

You know the saying, 'If in doubt, leave it out'. If something doesn't 'feel right' perhaps it is a warning.

A mild to general yoga class will generally aid the average backache and help the student feel pleasantly stretched and 'good'.

# SECTION 1

## WARM-UPS, GENERAL POSTURES AND TWISTS

### SIDE ROLLS

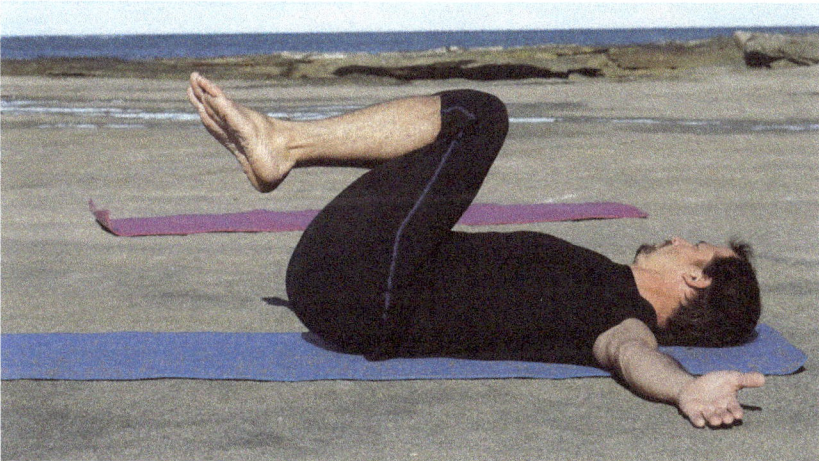

Lie on your back, arms stretched out at shoulder level.

If you have the palms facing up rather than down, the shoulder blades can ease further onto the mat and you may find it more relaxing.

Having the palms down will give you more grip to control the movement. See which feels appropriate for your body.

Bring the knees up to the chest and rock the hips from side to side for some seconds. Use this time to slow down the breath. Breathe in, when your knees are central, breathe out, as you ease them to the left or right.

As your knees go one way, let your head turn to look over the *opposite* shoulder. After 30-60 seconds come back to the centre with your knees over your chest. Arms still out at shoulder level.

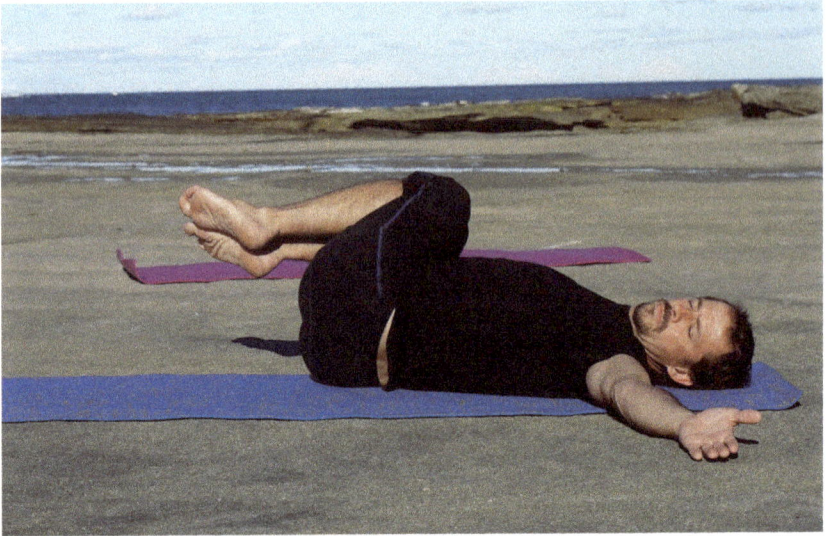

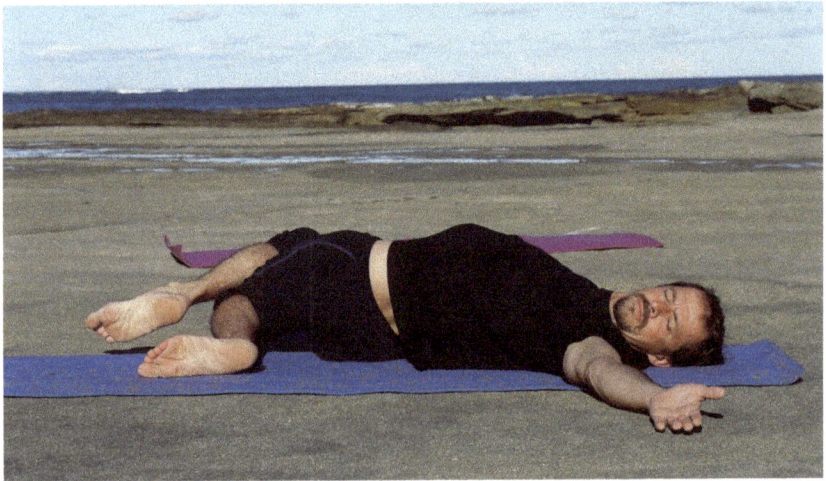

Take a deep breath in. As you breathe out, take the legs to the right side, keeping the left arm out and looking over your left arm. Head one way - body the other. Finally, hold down the outer edge of the top leg, the left leg, with your right hand. Take a few deep breaths in and out through the nose while in this position. Then breathe in and come back to the centre position, knees above your chest.

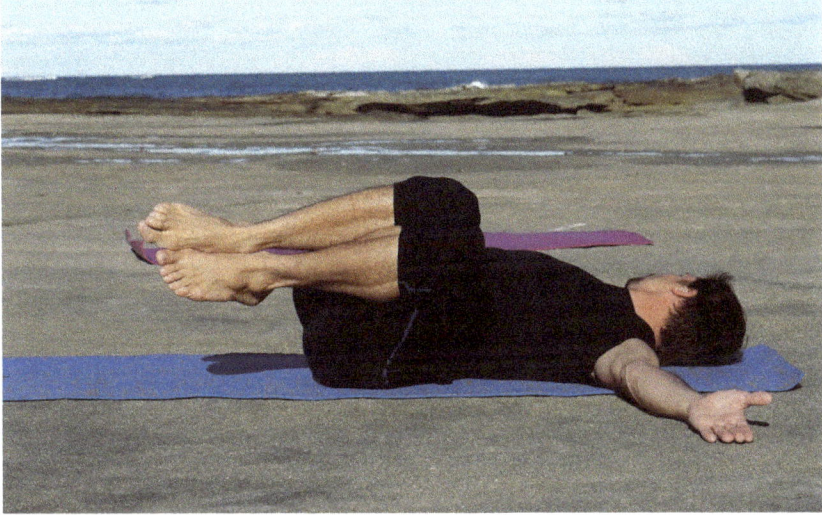

Now breathe out to the left side. Keep the right arm and hand stretched out and look over your right shoulder towards your hand. Deep breathing in and out through the nose. Finally, hold your legs down with your left hand on the outside of the top (your right) leg, near the knee, to enhance the stretch.

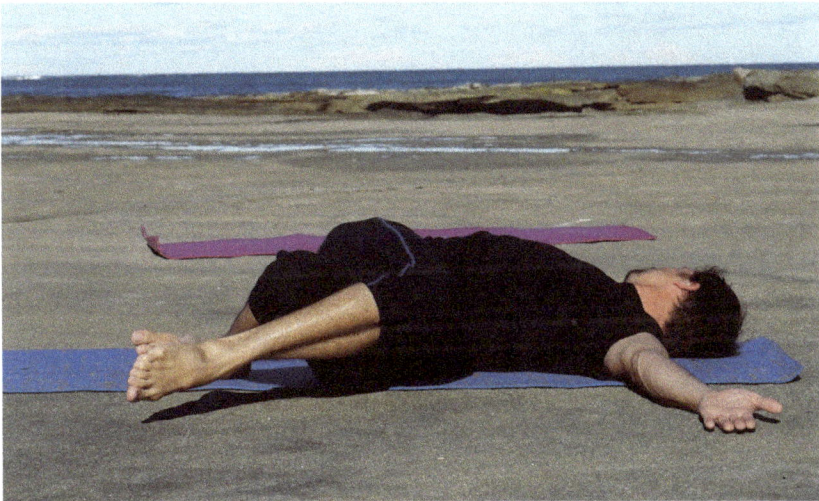

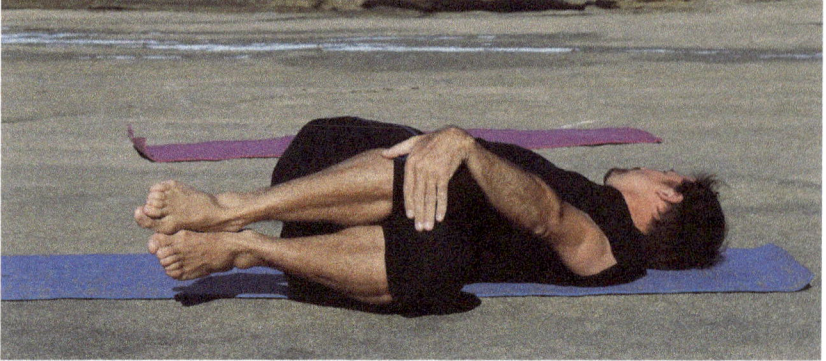

Breathe in and come back to centre position. Lower the legs down to the mat and relax.

## WIND RELIEVING POSE - PAVANMUKTASANA

Lie on your back with the legs straight up. Breathe in; as you breathe out, bring the knees into your chest.

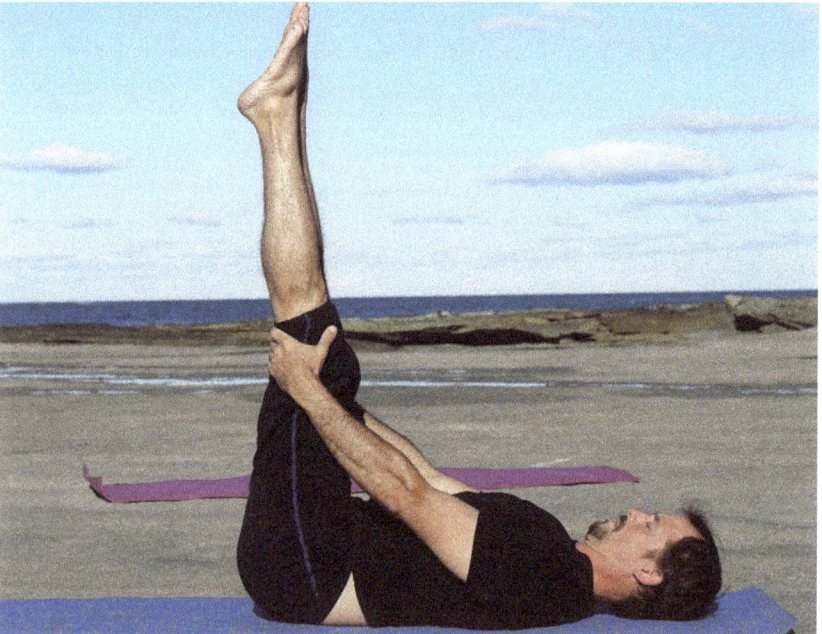

This movement aims to relieve flatulence. That is, it moves air around and is likely to cause it to come out - not negate it!

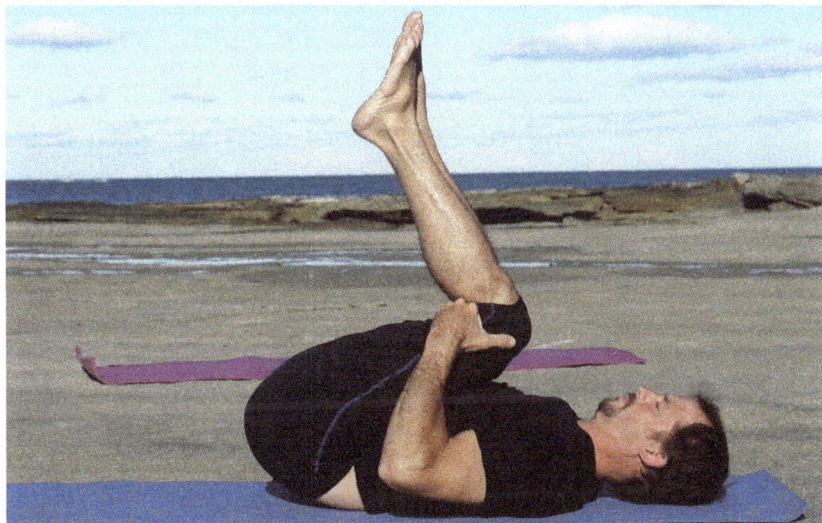

It also helps proper elimination and relieves tiredness in the legs.

## THE BRIDGE - SETU BANDHA SARVANGASANA

Lie on your back with your knees up, feet up to your buttocks. Have the feet hip distance apart on the floor, knees in line with your heels.

Press down with the inside of your arms and hands, the balls and heels of your feet, and slowly lift your lower back, hips, middle and upper back off the floor, so that you are resting on your shoulders and feet.

Gently ease the shoulder blades inwards; the chin should touch the chest without bringing the chin down.

Both the thighs should be parallel to each other and to the floor. Have your knees no wider than your hip width. Don't let the legs relax and fall outwards. The buttocks and thighs are to be active.

This beginning posture helps strengthen the hips, lower back muscles and legs. It also opens the chest.

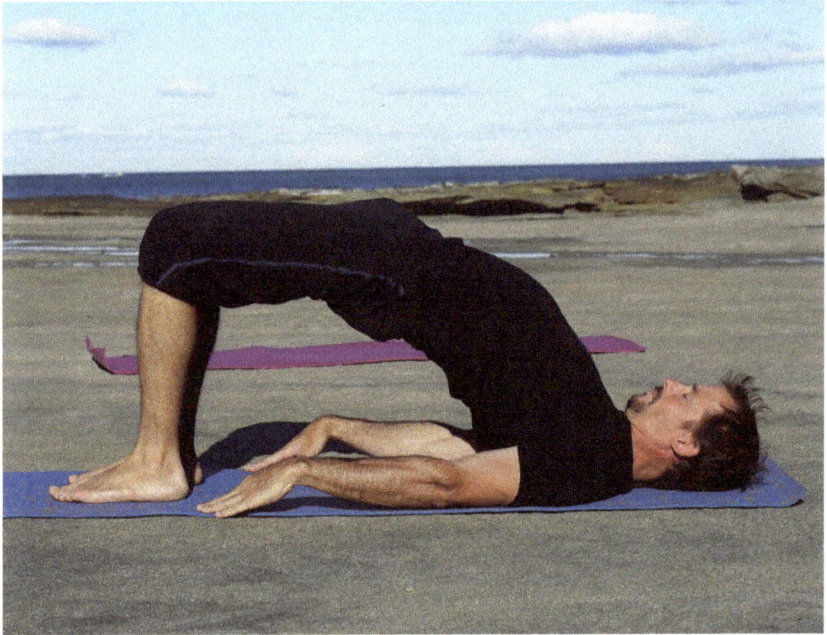

Take a few slow, deep breaths in and out while holding the posture, with your forearms into the mat. Alternatively, you could interlace the fingers stretching the arms towards your feet and push the hands down on the floor to lift the torso a little higher.

If more comfortable, place your hands on the back of your hips to support your back and help push up your hips. After a few deep breaths, gently lower the shoulder blades, followed by the rest of the body.

Bring the knees to the chest and roll around hugging your knees to massage the back. Think of a clock hand. Rock down the left side of your back, across the coccyx, up the right side and across the shoulder blades, several times, then reverse the order, rolling anti-clockwise.

NOTE: For a stronger stretch, the supported bridge, using a block, can be attempted after the body is warmed up, generally towards the end of your session. For this reason, the pose will be repeated in Section 4, including instructions for stretching out on a block.

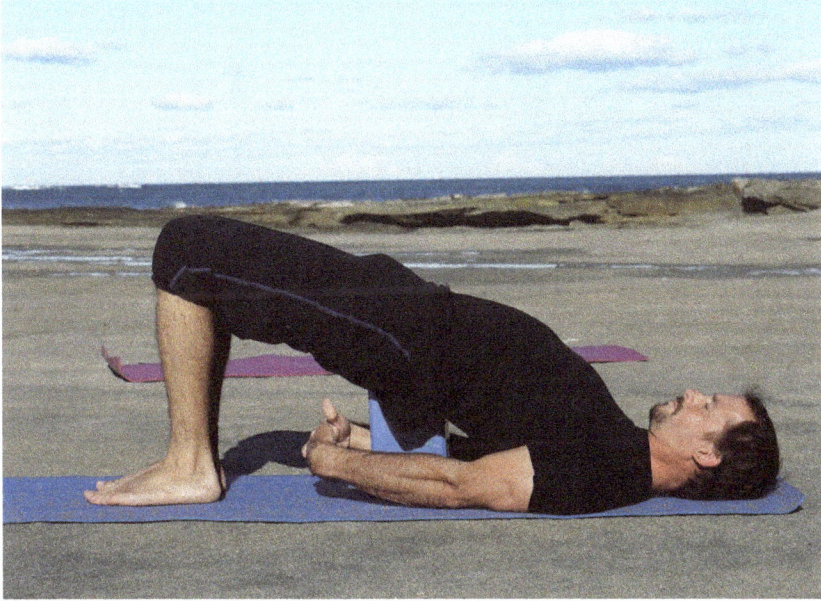

When using a block, you will have the block handy by the side of your body. Keep your back on the mat. Bend the knees and place the feet flat on the floor to lift the hips up supporting yourself with your arms on the mat, as the first posture. Once the hips are lifted, take the block the tall-way up, if the flexibility of your spine permits, and, place the block under the sacrum - the last few vertebrae of the spine before the coccyx or tailbone.

Some students may need to come slightly up on the toes for a few seconds to facilitate placement of the block, but if this applies to you, ensure once the block is in place, that the feet are firmly planted down again. The feet should be flat for stability. Keep the thighs active.

Remove the block and gently lower the back to the mat. For a stronger stretch on the block, see Section 4, where, if stable, you can walk your legs out into a straight line. After the bridge pose using a block, particularly, make sure you bring your knees to your chest and gently rock around on the back to massage it, as described earlier. Do this for 30 seconds. Now rock yourself up into a sitting position. This can be done by crossing the ankles, holding onto your big toes; rocking backwards and forwards then up into a cross-legged sitting position.

Once sitting, have the back straight, close the eyes and take a few deep breaths. Be aware of the body and the breath in and out.

## STAR POSE - BADDHAKONASANA

Sit on the mat with the knees out wide and bring the soles of the feet together.

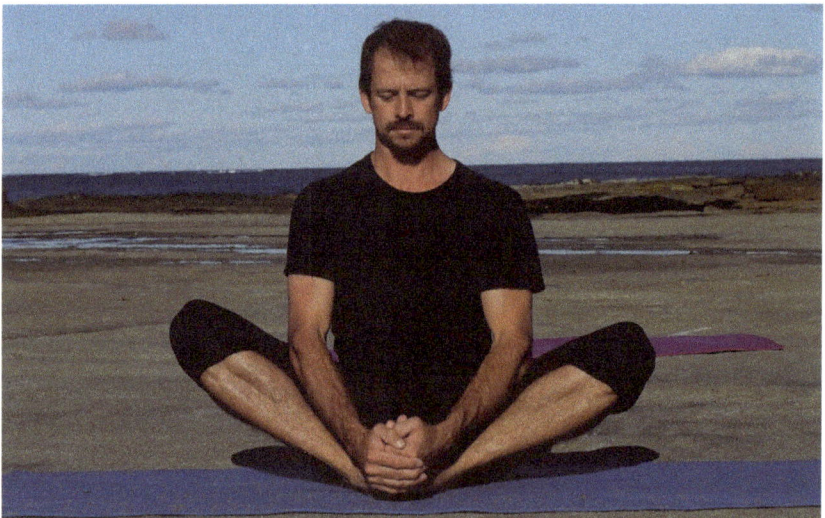

To warm up: hold your feet with your hands and rock from your right to your left.

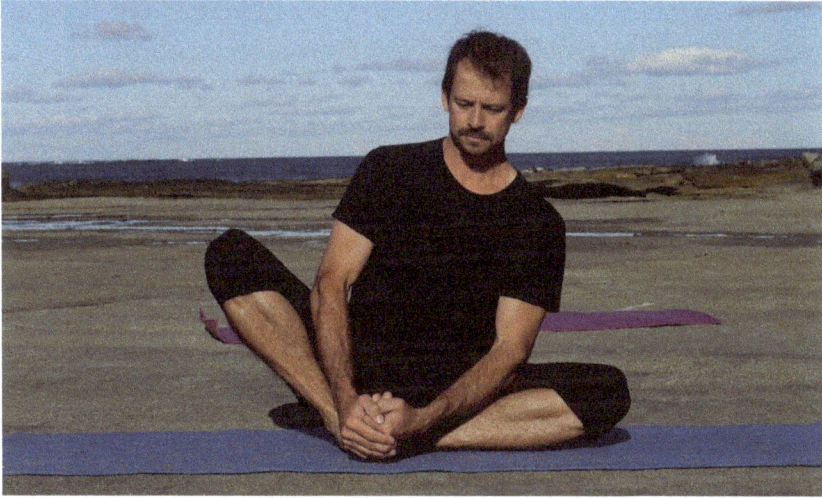

You can use your forearms to stretch the legs further down towards the floor. Over time, the knees will sink lower. Now come back to central position.

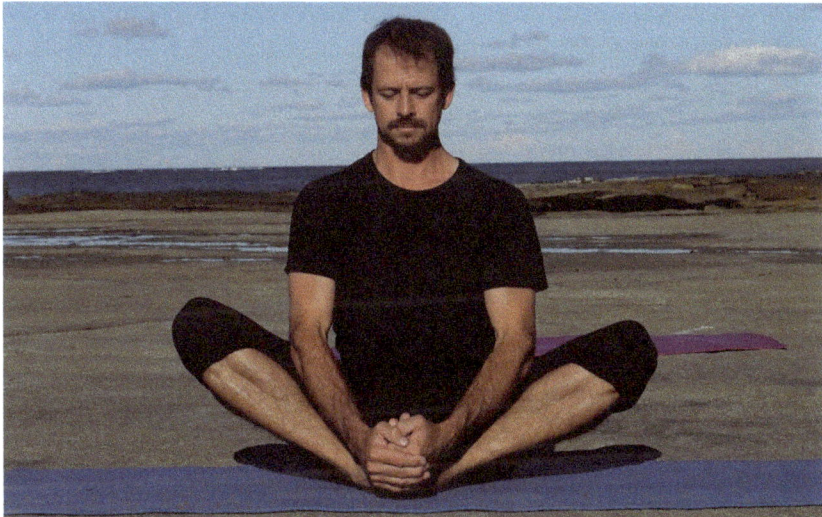

Grasping your feet firmly, pull them closer into the groin. Both heels should touch the groin. Sit right up on the sitting bones.

Take a deep breath in then ease your thighs to the floor as you breathe out. Keep stretching the spine upwards.

This posture, and the following extension, limbers the lower back and hips.

For women, it can make childbirth easier so is a good posture during pregnancy (*without* the following extension). It stretches the inner thigh muscles.

To extend from this posture, exhale slowly bringing your forehead as near to the feet as is comfortable. Draw the stomach in as you sink forward. Bring the forearms outside the shins.

## JUST STRETCHING

Sit cross-legged the easiest way for you. Stretch both arms up then keeping a long back, stretch forward from the lower body and place the tips of the forefinger and middle finger on the floor in front of you, arms straight. Keep the neck long and not bent up or down. Simply look at the ground about a metre in front of you. Breathe in and then as you breathe out, walk the hands to the right side, keeping the left buttock down.

Breathe in and come back to the centre. Breathe out again and walk your hands to the left side, keeping the right buttock down. Now breathe in and stretch up again, then breathe out and lower the arms by your sides.

Reverse the way your legs are crossed. This no doubt will be the less natural way for you to cross your legs. Repeat the stretches in the same way as you did when your legs were crossed the other way.

Now sit up into a comfortable cross-legged position.

## SHOULDER ROLLS

Bring your fingertips to your shoulders - right hand on right shoulder, left on left.

Bring the elbows up by the side of your face and ears, elbows pointing out in front of your forehead, and breathe in. Hold the breath as you stretch the elbows out at the sides and back and breathe out as you bring them forward and in across your chest. Bring them up again, breathing in, and keep repeating until you have done this at least three times.

Now, hands still on your shoulders, reverse the order: bring the shoulder blades together as you breathe in, stretching the elbows back behind the bottom ribs; hold the breath as you bring the elbows up like wings at shoulder level, and breathe out as you bring them in across your chest. Repeat three times.

## BREATHING

To relax the body, just close your eyes and take some deep breaths in and out through the nose. Make your exhalation longer than the inhalation. Breathe into the whole diaphragm.

If possible, try and do this in front of a mirror because your shoulders should not move up and down. Your upper chest should be still. Think of a golden balloon in front of your waist, extending down to your belly and up to your chest.

When you breathe in, this balloon, and your lungs beneath it, must fill with air and therefore the whole abdominal wall is pushed out and expands. When you breathe out, the balloon goes down, as does your whole abdominal wall.

Think of breathing into the very bottom of your lungs first, then the middle part. Air flows almost passively into the top part without you needing to puff out the top of your chest. If air only goes into the small upper part of the lungs, and you never breathe deeply enough to fill the whole lungs, this shallow breathing is likely to cause stress. You will breathe naturally, the correct way, when relaxing, for example, read-ing a book.

As a general rule, when practising yoga, postures that lift and open the chest are done with an inhalation, and postures which fold forward and close the chest require an exhalation with the fold. Twists are completed on the exhalation.

Although guidelines are given to hold a pose for a certain number of breaths or seconds, do what is comfortable or appropriate for you.

*FOR SPECIFIC BREATHING EXERCISES, SEE SECTION 7 FOLLOWING THE END OF THE POSTURES.*

## FROM THE FOLLOWING POSTURES

After practising the gentle postures shown, in each session, pick: a forward stretch, a back stretch, a spinal twist, some cat and dog postures, salute to the sun, some standing stretches, a balance, a restful posture, and, if possible, a shoulder stand or half shoulder stand followed by a fish posture.

If unsure due to injury or back issue, check with a doctor or physiotherapist.

Please note that during the time of menstruation females should not invert the body. In such a case, and if you are unable to do a shoulder stand for other reasons, simply rest with your back on your mat and elevate the legs straight up into the candle position. Alternatively, see 'LEGS UP THE WALL' position in Section 6, where the back is also kept on the mat.

Your body and spine permitting, always follow a shoulder stand with a fish posture. After a bridge or strong back bend, bring the knees up to the chest. After forward facing backbend postures, such as cobra, locust and boat, slide back onto your heels and lower the head to the floor by your knees into a child posture.

## FORWARD STRETCH FOR THE LOWER BACK

This is for your lower back, and not intended to be the full yoga posture PASCHIMOTTASANA, where the body is lowered to the legs. The above can be used as a warm-up before PASCHIMOTTASANA, which is addressed in Section 4.

Sit with your legs out in front of you and back straight. Walk each buttock back, one-two, to position yourself towards the front of the sitting bones.

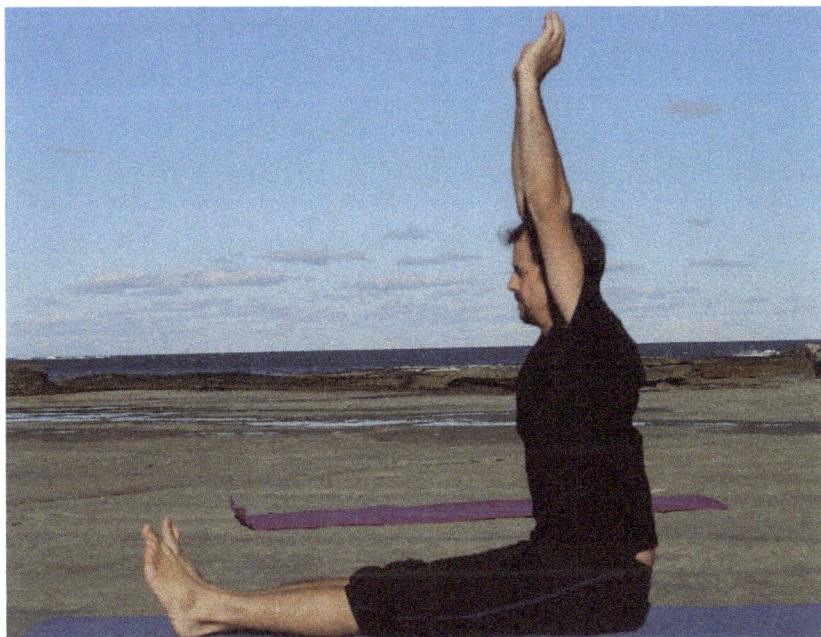

Breathe in and stretch the arms up either side of your ears. Breathe out and stretch forward slightly from the hip joints, not from the waist. Reach towards your toes, keeping the back as long and straight as possible. It doesn't matter if you can't reach the toes, just keep the arms out in front, reaching forward for a few seconds.

Keep the head upright and gaze beyond your toes.

On each exhalation stretch and extend forward without letting your head or chest drop forward.

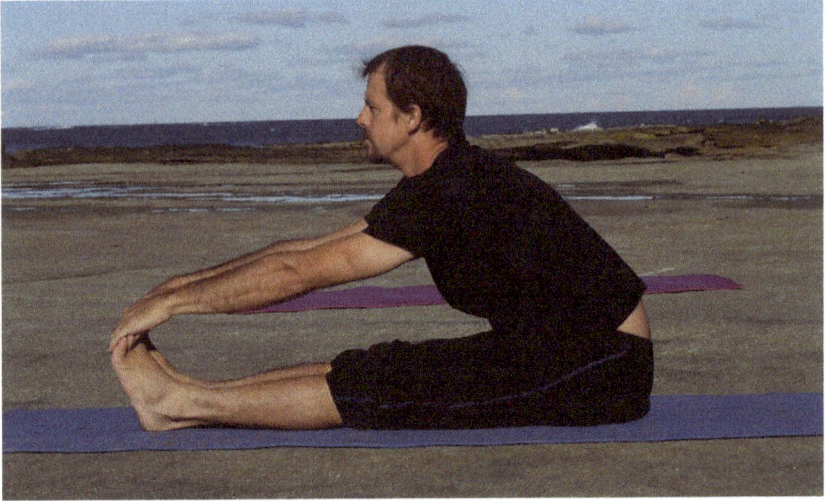

Keep the back as straight as you can, even though the whole back will be slightly forward leaning.

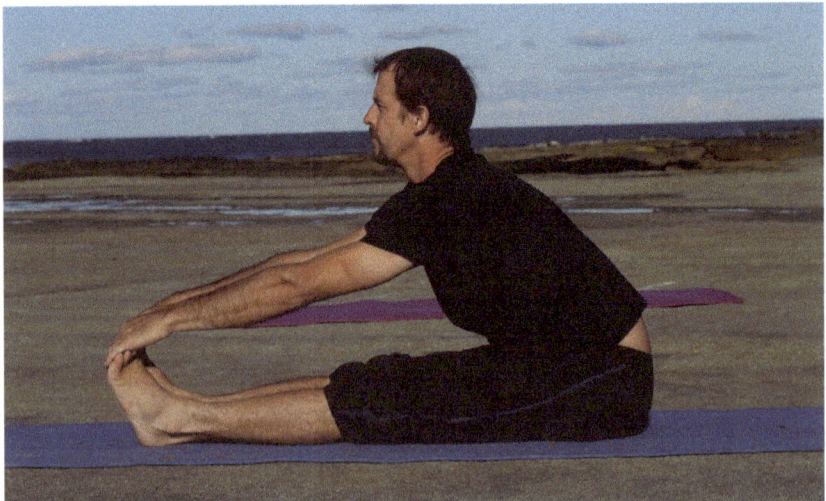

After stretching for a few seconds, rest your hands on the toes or wherever they reach. Soften the knees more if your calves hurt.

Maintain for a few more seconds breathing in and out freely. Breathe in, stretch up again, and breathe out, lower your hands by your sides.

## BACK STRETCH

Sit with your legs straight out in front of you. Back straight. Clasp your hands behind your back, breathe in and pull the shoulder blades together. Hold. Breathe out and relax.

## SIMPLE SPINAL TWISTS

While sitting with your legs out, here's a simple spinal twist for energy.

Breathe in, and as you breathe out, take your right hand across the front of your body and slip the hand under the left knee. Place the left hand behind you and press the heel of the hand into the floor.

Look over your left shoulder.

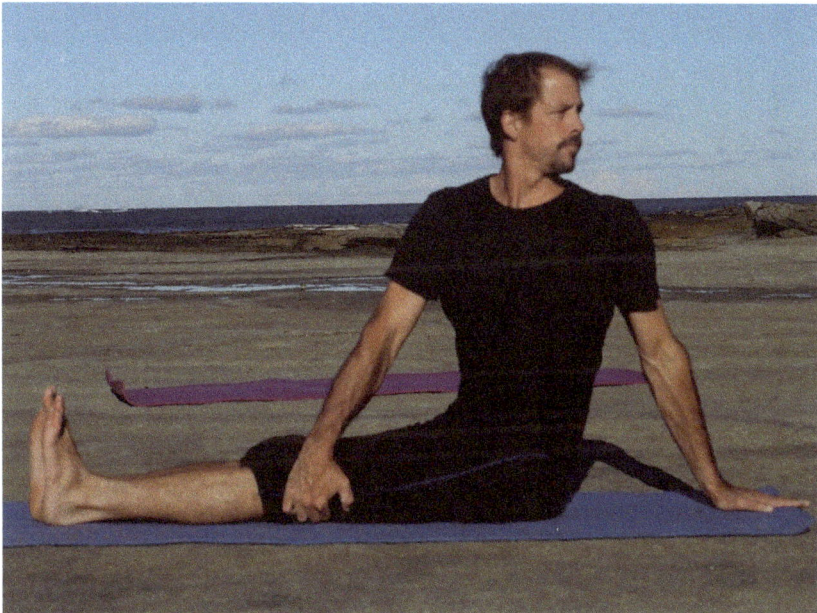

Hold the posture and deep breathe in and out for several seconds. Breathe in, and as you breathe out, swing the left hand over the front of the body to slip the hand under the right knee.

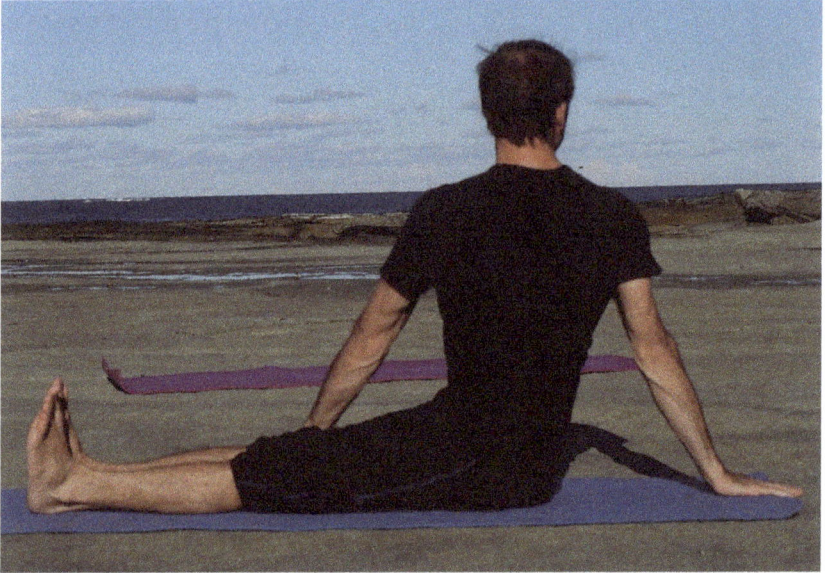

Place the right hand behind you and look over the right shoulder. Hold for a few seconds breathing slowly and evenly.

Finally, breathe in, and as you breathe out, bring your arms back by your sides, in preparation for the wide-angle seated forward bend - UPAVISTHA KONASANA.

The following pose is good preparation for most seated forward bends, twists, and the wide-leg standing poses.

## WIDE-ANGLE SEATED FORWARD BEND - UPAVISTHA KONASANA

Have the legs wide apart. If there's discomfort having the legs wide, a folded blanket can be used under the coccyx and back part of the buttocks. Another option is to roll a little section of your mat under the base of the spine.

Sit up straight. Press the thighs into the floor, the kneecaps pointing upwards.

Breathe in and stretch your arms up. Pre-posture stretch.

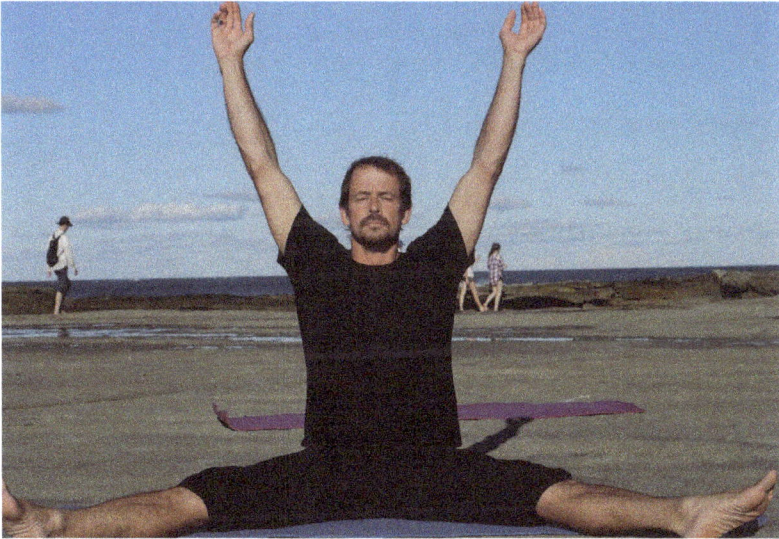

Breathe out and slide the arms down in between the legs, moving forward from the hips, or simply slide the arms forward (without stretching up) as you extend from the hips. Stretching up first may help you to lengthen through the back.

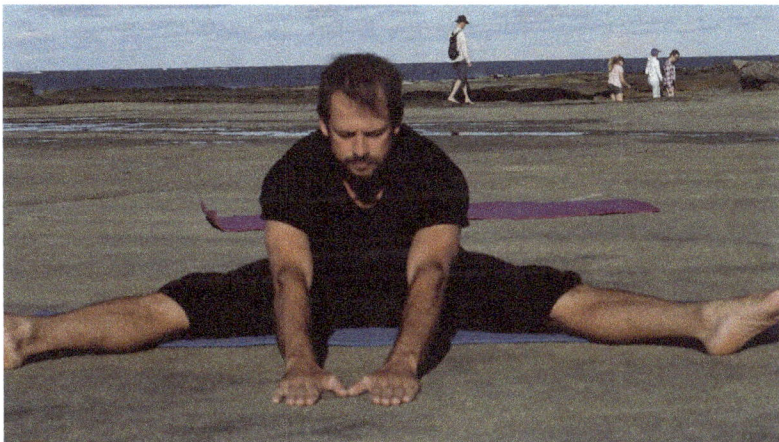

Sit up straight again. On your next exhalation, lean forward from the hips and stretch towards your toes, keeping a long, straight back. Go as far as you can without bending, then grasp the big toes with the index and middle fingers.

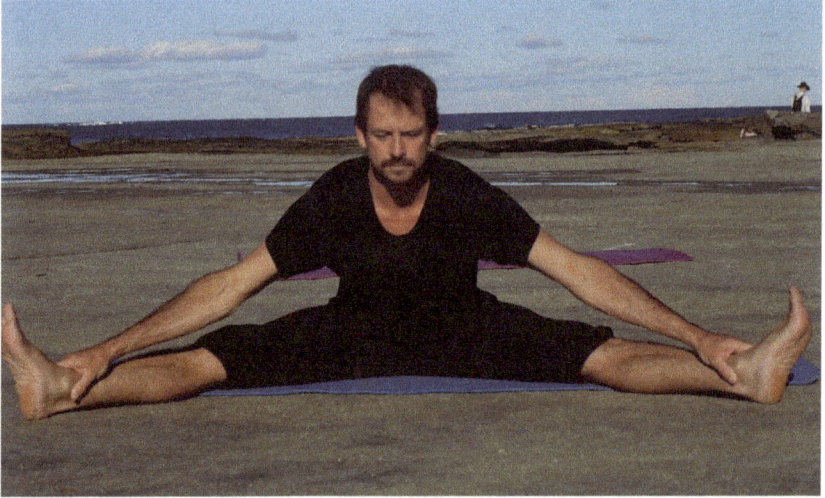

If you can't reach the toes, grasp the calves and stretch as far as the back allows. *If* you're able to extend forward more from the hips, vary this posture thus:

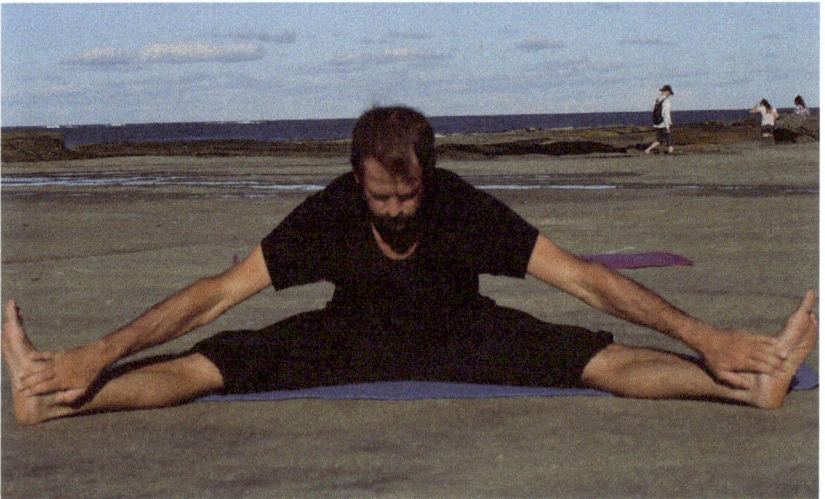

On an exhalation, slide the hands back to the floor between the legs; at the same time, stretch from the hips and lower the torso to the floor.

Some students may need to use cushions and lower the body to them. Bend the elbows outwards as your torso lowers to the cushion or floor.

Whether stretching to grasp your toes, body to the floor, or to rest the chest on a cushion, breathe in and come up, stretching the arms above your head. Breathe out, lower the hands down by your side.

From this wide legged position, it is easy to do another variation of a simple spinal twist.

From a sitting position, breathe in, then as you breathe out, take your right arm down the inside of your body close to the diaphragm. Take your left arm behind the mid-line of your body, with the heel of the back hand pressed into the mat about 10 - 20 centimetres away from your body. Hold for a few breaths.

With your upper arm against the diaphragm, be aware of the breath.

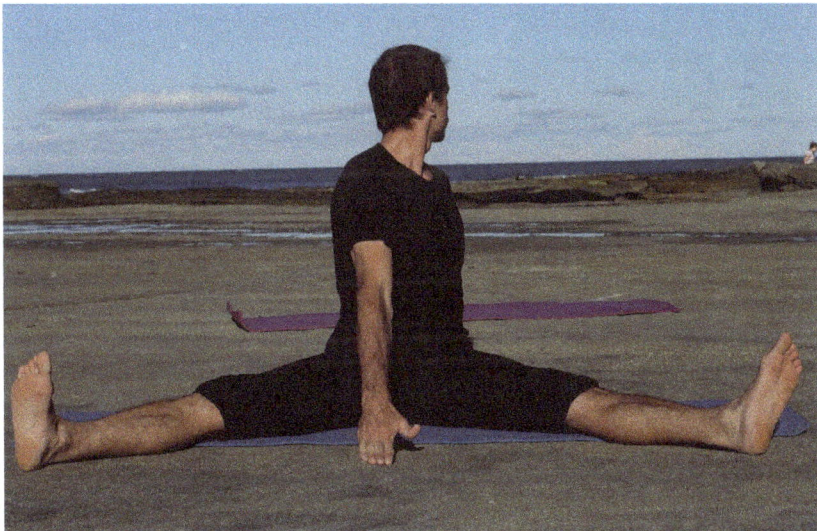

As you breathe in, the diaphragm extends out towards your arm as the lungs expand, as you breathe out, it sinks back to the body, away from your arm.

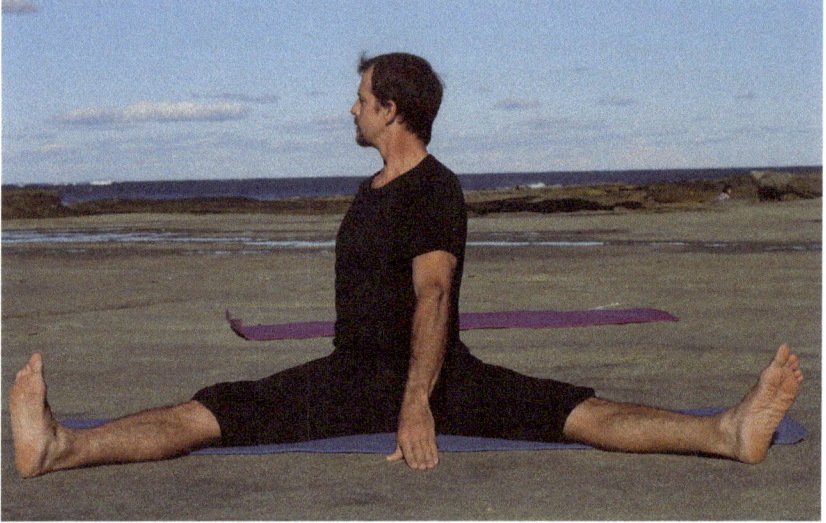

Reverse, with the left arm in front, the right behind. Breathe in and come back to a central position, your arms by your sides. What next?

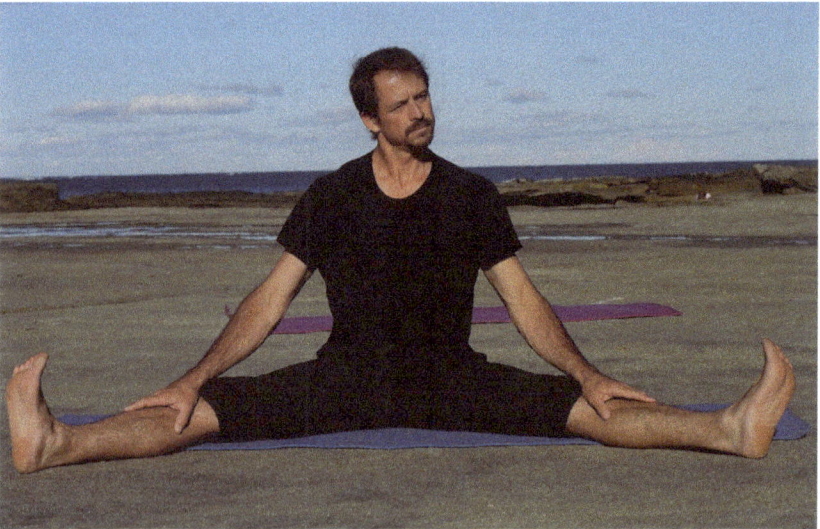

Bring the legs together, stretched out in front of you on the mat, in preparation for the SPINAL TWIST - ARDA MATSYENDRASANA.

## SPINAL TWIST - ARDA MATSYENDRASANA

There are a few variations of the spinal twist. The following postures are commonly practised in general classes.

Sit up straight with your legs *together* out in front of your body. Bend the right leg over the left. Begin by simply hugging the right knee with your LEFT arm and hand so that the knee is close to your left armpit.

Breathe in and take the right hand behind the spine a few centimetres away from the body. Press down with the heel of the hand.

Look over your right shoulder.

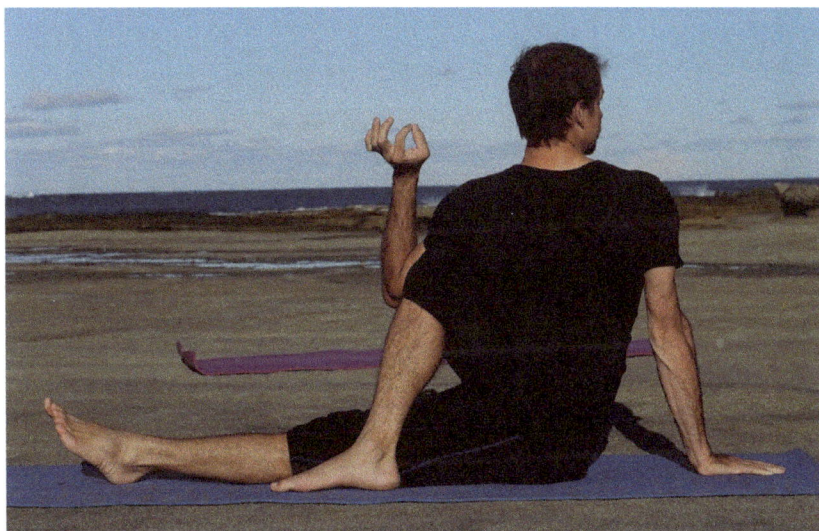

The above picture shows a more advanced hold where the left elbow is pressed against the outside of the right knee rather than wrapping around it, and with the thumb and finger closed in a mudra. (See mudras, further on in this section).

This can also be done with the palm facing out, without joining the thumb and index finger in a mudra. If trying either of these versions, take care not to strain the area around the shoulder blade. Not recommended for those with shorter arms or upper body inflexibility.

Press down with the heel of the hand more if you wish to strengthen the twist. Be aware of the breath again: as you breathe in, the diaphragm moves out and the lungs fill with air. Feel the movement against the inside of your right thigh. As you breathe out, the diaphragm falls back to the spine.

Now the left side: Sit up straight with your legs out in front of your body. Bend the left leg over the right. Hug the knee with your RIGHT arm. Breathe in and take the left hand behind the spine. Look over your left shoulder.

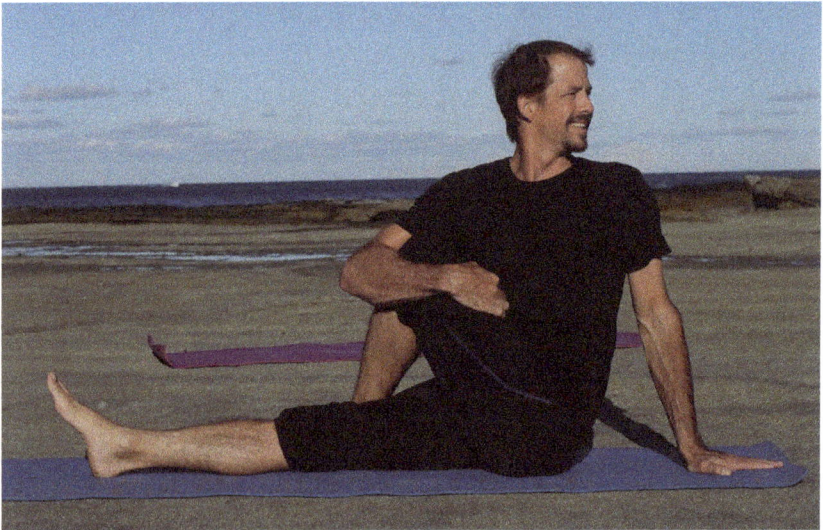

If your arms and shoulders are flexible, try the elbow pressed into the outside of the knee, either with the palm facing forward or the forefinger and thumb closing together in a circle, making the GYAN mudra.

After a few seconds release the leg and resume a sitting posture.

### *On Fingers and Thumbs:*

A very brief summary on fingers and thumbs and one of the more common hand mudras: GYAN MUDRA.

The **little finger** represents earth element, the energy centre corresponding to the base of the spine, MOOLADHARA CHAKRA (energy centre) - area of the gonads.

The **ring finger** represents the water and corresponds to the centre situated between the hips, SWADHISTHANA CHAKRA. It is the area associated with the suprarenal glands (Adrenals).

The **middle finger** represents the solar plexus, or sun centre at the centre of the body. It corresponds to the element of fire and is known as MANIPURA CHAKRA. Its association is with the pancreas.

The **index finger** represents the heart centre which corresponds to air - ANAHATA CHAKRA. The endocrine gland is the thymus, above the heart.

The **thumb** symbolises that which is beyond the four physical elements, sometimes as depicted as space.

In joining the thumb and the finger you are joining your highest element, air, by way of the heart, to the universe. It is a meditative stance to bring you more in tune with your higher self, which you might call your God consciousness. It is known as the GYAN MUDRA and helps to improve your concentration and sharpen your memory.

While it is used in some postures, it is commonly used when sitting in meditation at the end of a class. See under meditation towards the end of the book.

## SPINAL TWIST - ARDA MATSYENDRASANA (BENT LEG VERSION)

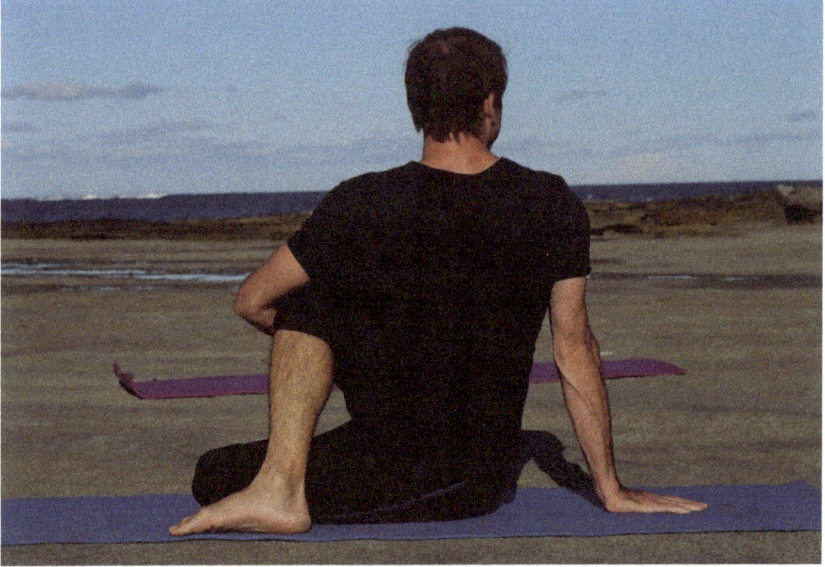

Sit with your legs out in front of you as for the previous pose.

Now bend the left leg and place the heel of the left foot beside the right hip.

Place the right leg up and over, so that the knee is facing up and the foot is in line with the left knee.

Hug the right knee close to your body with the left arm. Have your right arm behind you, towards the mid-line of your body and press down with the heel of the hand. Look over your right shoulder.

*Variations:*

Slide the left arm OUTSIDE the right knee, elbow bent; forearm and palm facing outwards, as in the former, long-legged posture.

Alternatively, slide the RIGHT arm down the inner right leg. Grasp the ankle but look over the left shoulder with the left hand behind the body.

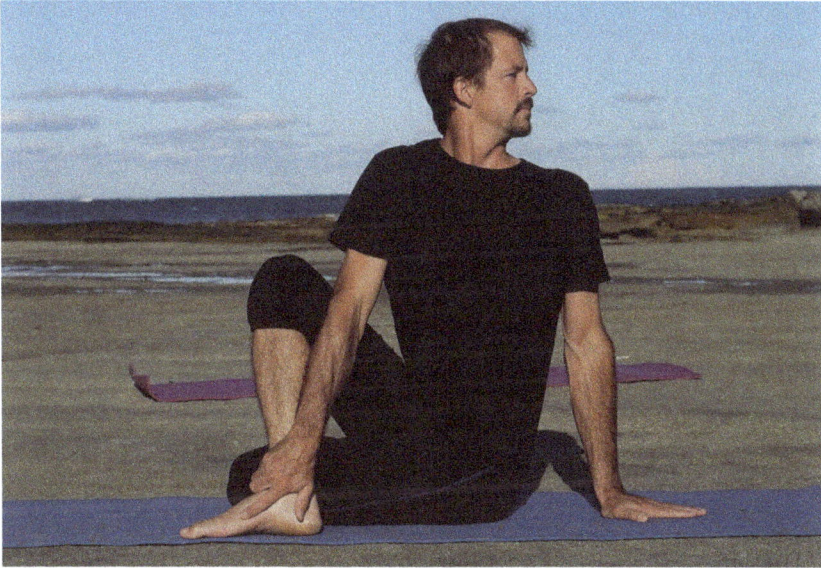

The legs have not moved in this third variation, you are simply varying the upper body twist.

Now do all that with the left leg up and over the right leg: Bend the right leg in with the toes towards the left hip. The left knee is facing up, crossed over the right with the toes in line with the right knee that is on the floor.

This time in most postures you will be twisting over your left shoulder, and either hugging your left knee with your right arm, or sliding the right elbow outside the left knee, forearm up and palm facing outwards, or with thumb and index finger joined in the hand mudra - GYAN MUDRA.

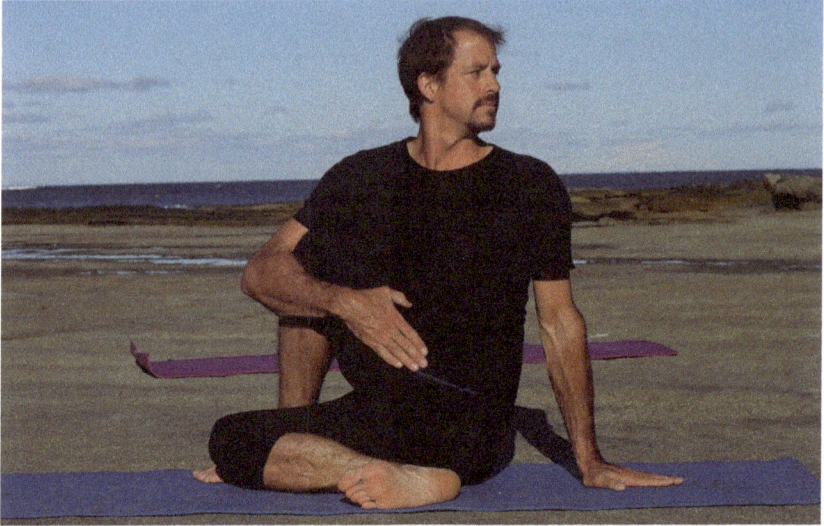

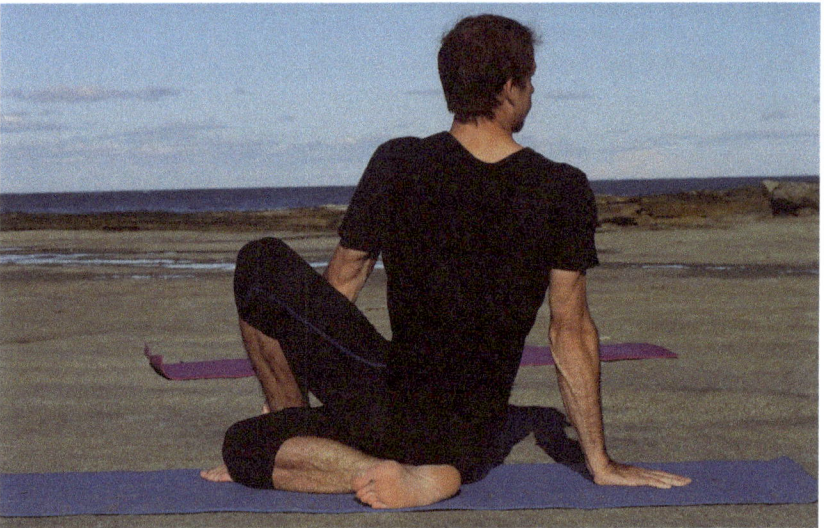

Finally, you might alter the upper body stance, slipping the left arm down inside the calf area to grasp the ankle. This time you will take your right arm behind you, the hand into the mat, to look over your right shoulder.

Breathe freely while you hold the posture for at least fifteen seconds.

To come out of the posture, come back into a cross-legged position or straighten the legs. This posture tones and/or massages many important organs and glands including the intestines, aiding the function of the body. It sends a flow of energy through the body.

## THE ARCHER - AKARNA DHANURASANA

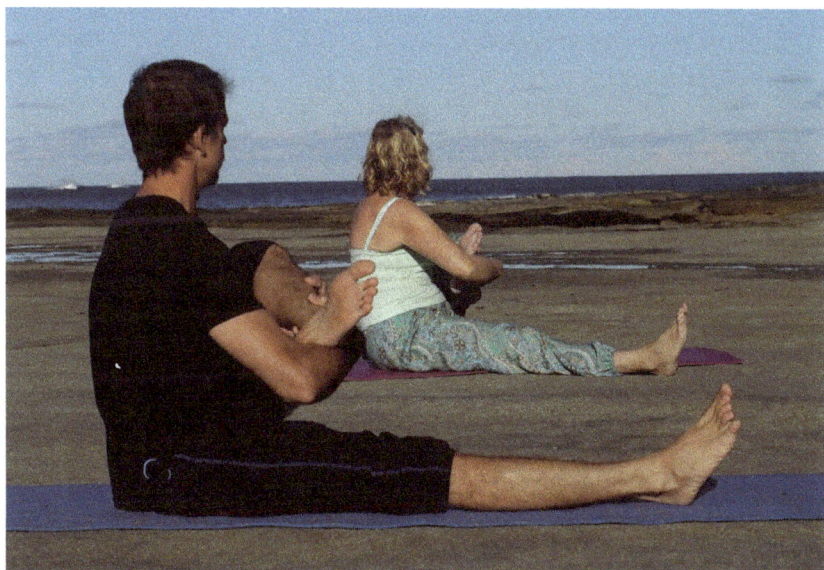

A great posture for the hip and pelvic region. There are many variations of the archer posture. This is a basic version.

Firstly, to warm up and ease the joints, sit with the right leg extended and the left leg bent in towards the body. Pick up the bent left leg behind the knee and rotate the ankle both ways, followed by the knee joint. Stretch your thigh and ease it from side to side from the pelvic joint. Now place the foot in the crease of the right elbow and the knee in the bend of the left elbow/forearm. Rock the bent knee from side to side as you might a baby.

Next, take the left big toe with the first two fingers of your right hand. Hook the fingers around the toe and draw the left foot up beside the right ear, as if drawing a bow to shoot an arrow. The elbow should be pointing back - behind the ear. If this can't be achieved yet, just hold the left foot in the right hand and raise the right elbow. Note: high elbow - high foot.

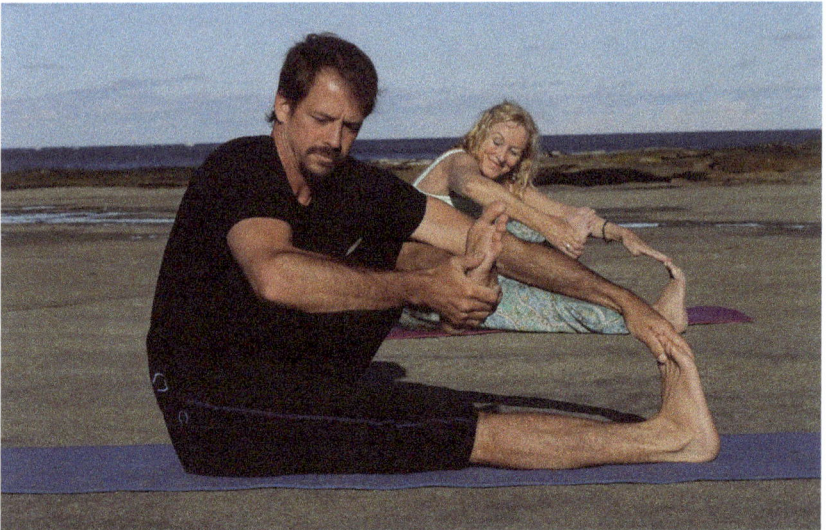

Whether you have hold of your toe or your foot with the right hand, stretch your *left* hand towards your right toes and grasp the big toe. Hold for ten seconds.

The archer is good for mobility of the hip joints and for the pelvic region. It should help to prevent the need for hip replacements.

For students who already have hip replacements (as with knee replacements) you may need to modify this posture somewhat. For example - keep both legs outstretched and just stretch to your toes.

Repeat on the other side, left leg out, right one bent in towards the body. Warm up by rocking the hip first as shown on the previous page, before taking the big toe of the right foot with the first two fingers of your left hand.

Draw the left elbow back behind your ear, or the alternative, hold your foot with the left hand and keep the left elbow high.

Stretch your right arm towards your extended left leg and hold the toes. Hold the position, deep breathing, for ten seconds.

## HEAD TO KNEE FORWARD BEND - JANUSIRASANA

This posture is best done with an empty stomach and bowel. Sit on the floor with the legs extended, then bend one leg in towards the body. Let's say you begin with the right leg out, the left in.

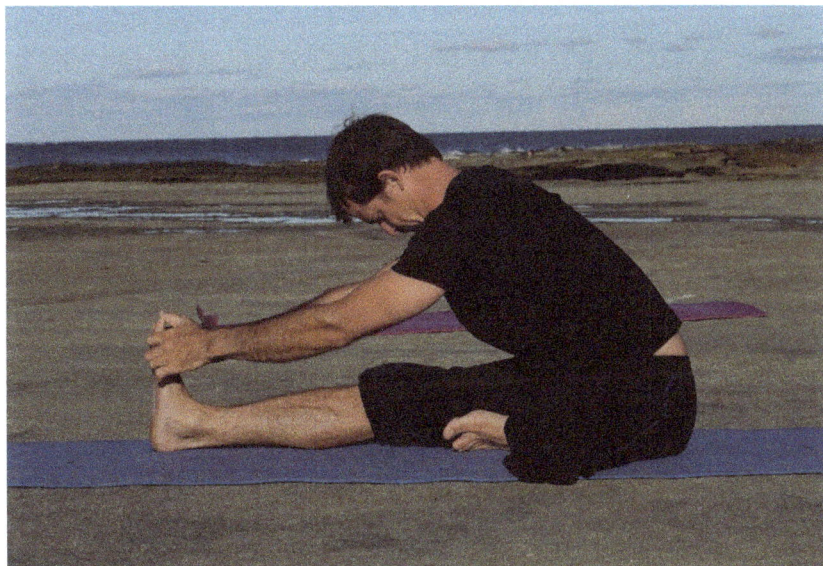

Ease the left knee down towards the mat and place the foot flat against the right thigh. Inhale and stretch the arms up, lengthening up from the hips.

Exhale and bend forward from the hips, then with both hands grasp the right foot and lower the chest and face towards the leg, or as near as possible. Keep a long back.

Avoid over-stretching if that means you would have to round the spine. Breathe deeply in and out. Maintain for several seconds, then release the pose. Breathe in and slowly come up to a sitting position. Now do the posture with the left leg out and the right leg bent in.

If you can't reach to your toes, rest the hands wherever you can on the knees, calves or ankles.

For the full extension: the body is extended to the thigh, with the hands grasping the extended foot. The chest and face rest on the leg. The elbows lower to the mat.

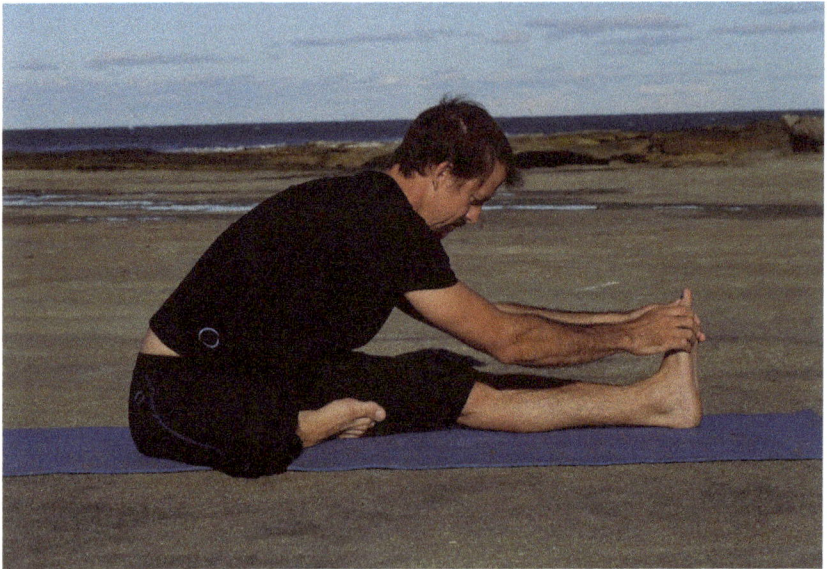

This posture tones the liver for digestion when done on the right side. It increases the blood and lymph from the spleen when done on the left.

JANUSIRASANA stimulates the kidneys. It has a calming effect, promotes elasticity and is good for all muscle groups.

## TWISTING HEAD TO KNEE POSTURE
## - PARIVRTTA SIRASANA - WARM UP

To warm up for the following posture: stretch out one leg and bend the other so that the instep rests on the floor by the top of the thigh/buttock on its own side.

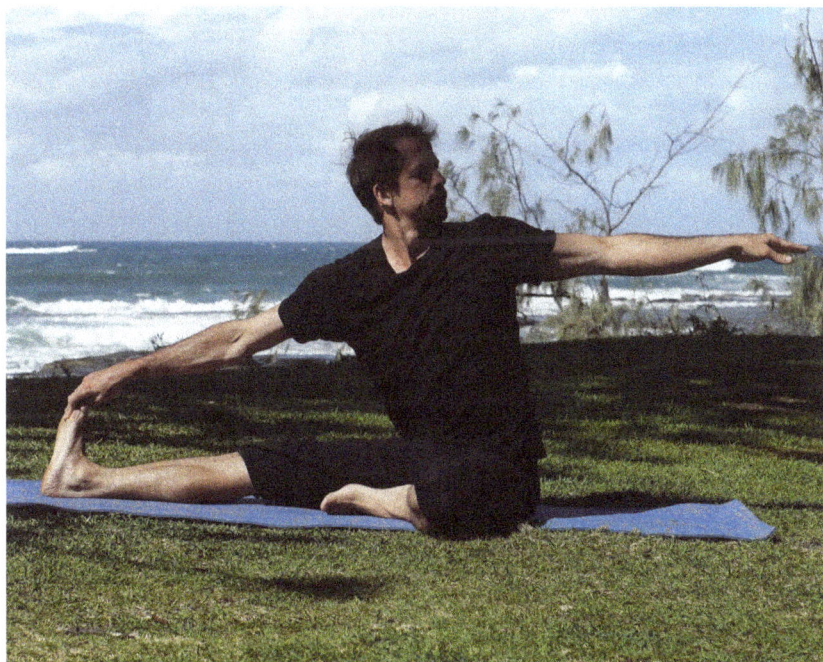

Reach for the toe of the outstretched leg with the arm of the same side. Stretch your other arm out at shoulder level and look at the thumb. Follow it with your gaze slightly behind the body, so that there is a slight twist in the ribs.

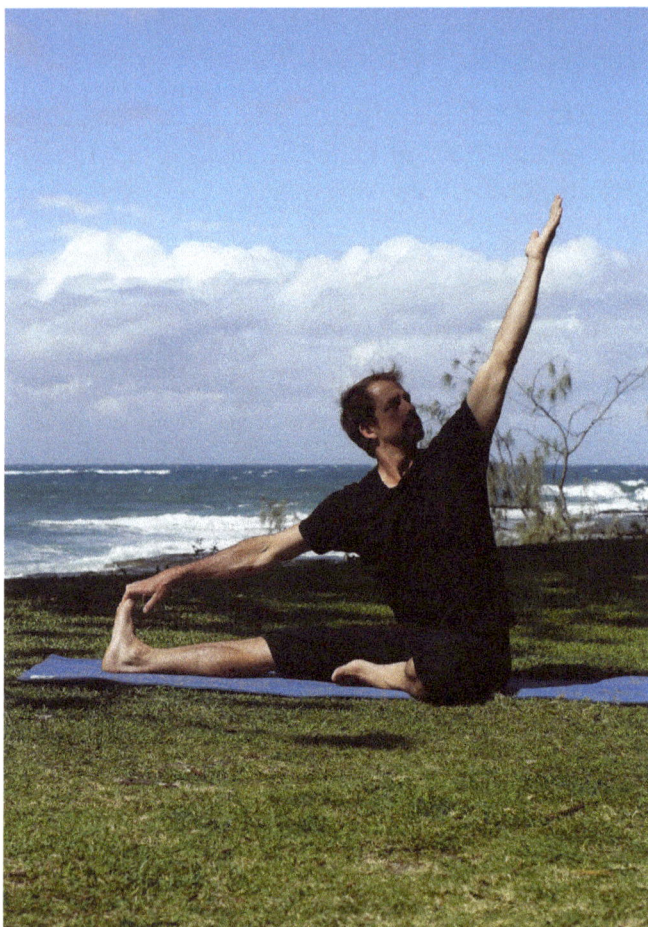

Now raise the arm you are stretching behind you, depicted here as the left arm. Bring it up with the underside of the arm close to your ear, then reach over your head, stretching your arm towards your extended right foot.

At the same time, lean the body towards the extended foot. Rest your raised hand on the wrist of the lower arm. Cross the wrists so that the thumbs are turned down and reach to clasp the foot on the outside of the extended right leg, with the crossed hands.

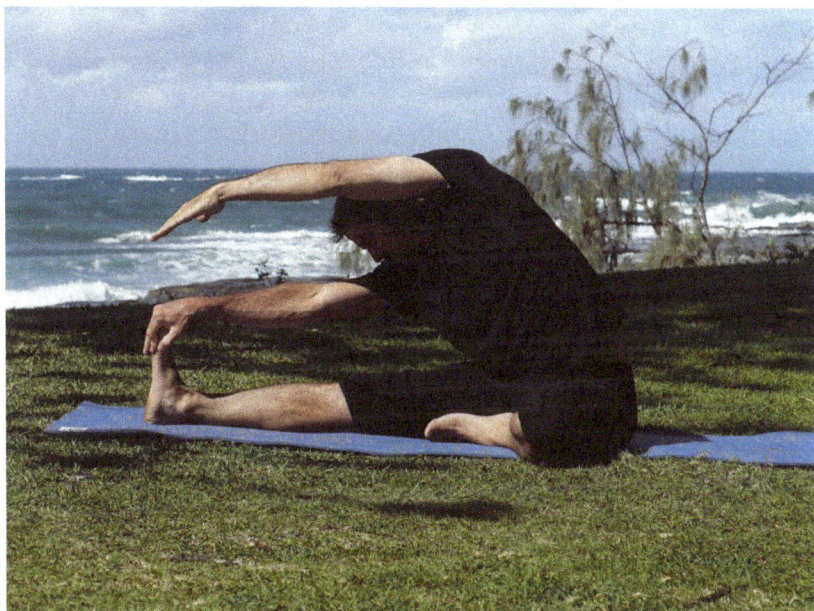

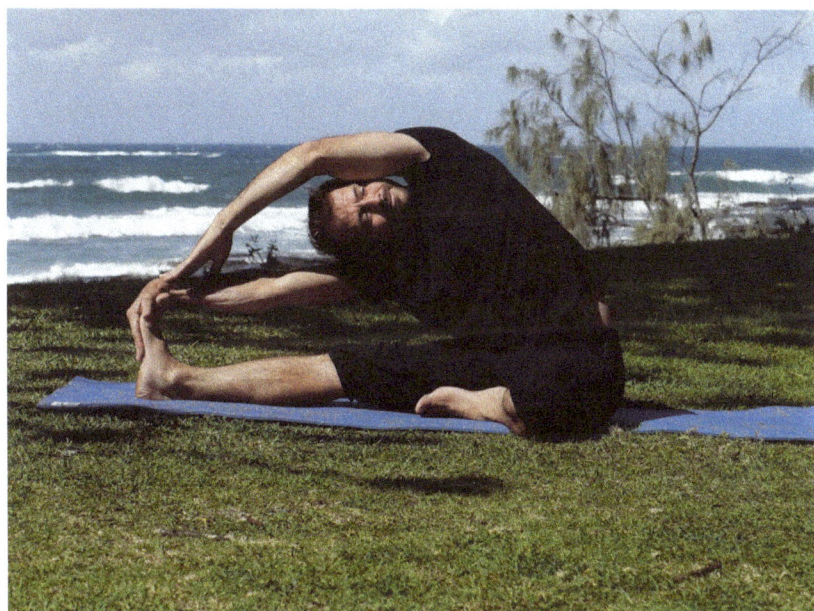

Stay for at least ten seconds, breathing in and out normally.

From this warm-up stretch, sit up straight with the legs as before: right leg out, with the left foot pressed against your right thigh towards the groin. Lean forward and down to press the back of your right shoulder against the inside of your right knee, lowering the trunk sideways towards the right leg.

Place the right forearm on the mat inside the right leg, palm up. Take the palm of your right hand to the inside edge of the foot and hold, with the thumb on the top of the foot and fingers on the sole.

Inhale and straighten the knee, if it isn't already. This will help you lengthen through the body. Twist your torso to the sky. Breathe in and take your left arm up and slightly back - behind your left ear. Stretch it over your head.

With your left arm over your head angled towards the extended right leg, take hold of the outside edge of the right foot. Twist the trunk upwards as if to look under the armpit, your head between your elbows. Widen the elbows to help twist the upper torso more.

As you spread the elbows, take the lower elbow to the floor. At the same time, lower the trunk further sideways to rest on the extended leg.

In tandem with this lowering of the body, continue to ease the ribs upwards. Angle your head to look towards the sky.

Hold for ten seconds, breathing deeply. Relax the twist and lower your body to the left /opposite side before sitting up.

Repeat on the other side. Re-align your legs so that now the left leg is stretched out and the right leg is bent in.

If you began with the warm-up posture, do the same on this side, before the full asana. Finally, after doing the posture to the left side, when coming out of the twist, lean your body to the right, before sitting up.

## THE CAT - MARJARIASANA and COW - BITILASANA

The cow is the arch, letting the waist drop down and looking up. The cat is the hump, breathing out, rounding the back and looking at the mat or thighs.

The posture is often just referred to as the cat. It is an easy posture, good for the whole back and should be used as a warm-up before attempting stronger postures.

Simply kneel with your knees under your hips and your hands under your shoulders. Keep the arms straight.

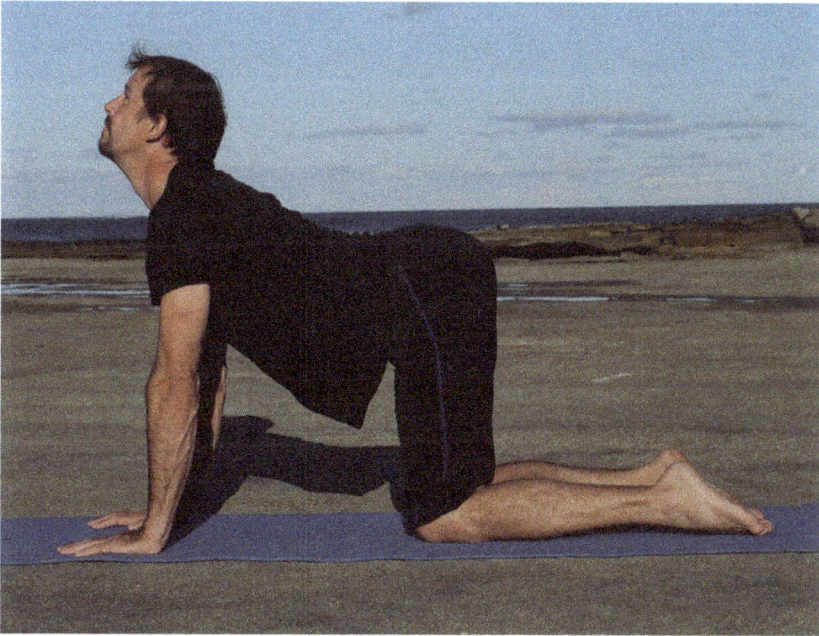

Breathe in slowly, arch the back by dipping the waist and look upwards. Let the stomach soften.

Now breathe out slowly and round the back, lifting the spine as much as possible as you make the cat-hump and look towards your thighs.

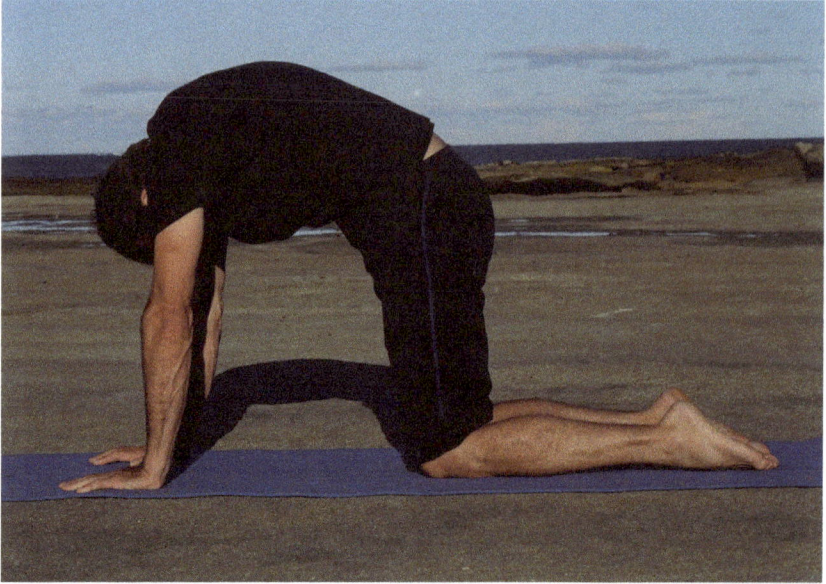

Let the exhalation when you hump, rounding the back, be at least the same length of time as the slow inhalation, when you arched the back.

*Unless* pregnant, you can also tighten the abdominals on the exhalation. If pregnant you may prefer not to let the waist drop into cow and stomach hang down. You might instead begin with a flat back like a table top. After the cat hump, rounding the back, go back to a table top.

The cat/cow is a mild back exercise which naturally adjusts the vertebrae and strengthens the back, pelvic and abdominal muscles. From cat hump you can walk the hands one hand forward and move the hips upwards into a 'dog stretch warm up'.

Think of bringing the hips up like a 'V' shape upside down. For this warm-up you can keep the knees relaxed and slightly bent.

## DOG STRETCH - ADHO MUKHA SVANASANA

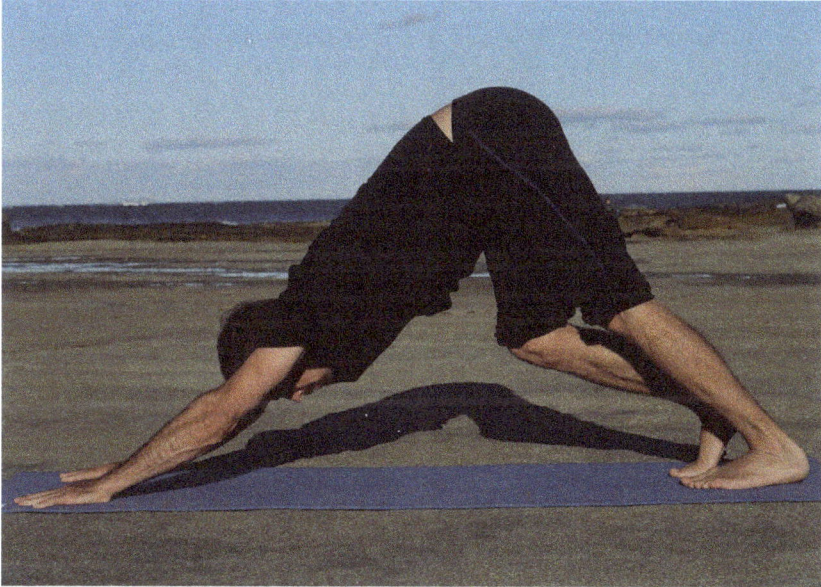

Push down with the heels of the hands and straighten the back. Now drop to the knees and push up again.

Then take the right heel to the floor keeping the left one bent, then the left heel to the floor softening or bending the right knee. Left, right, left, right. This is known as 'walking the dog'. Then come up onto the toes and stretch the ankles. Next, aim to get the heels down to the floor, but don't strain.

Have the space between your hands the same distance as the space between your feet.

For the full dog stretch, lift your hips as high as possible, if they aren't already, with the back straight, and take the head between straight arms - as if aiming for your knees. Flatten across the shoulder muscles.

This pose is repeated later as part of SURYA NAMA-SKAR: salute to the sun.

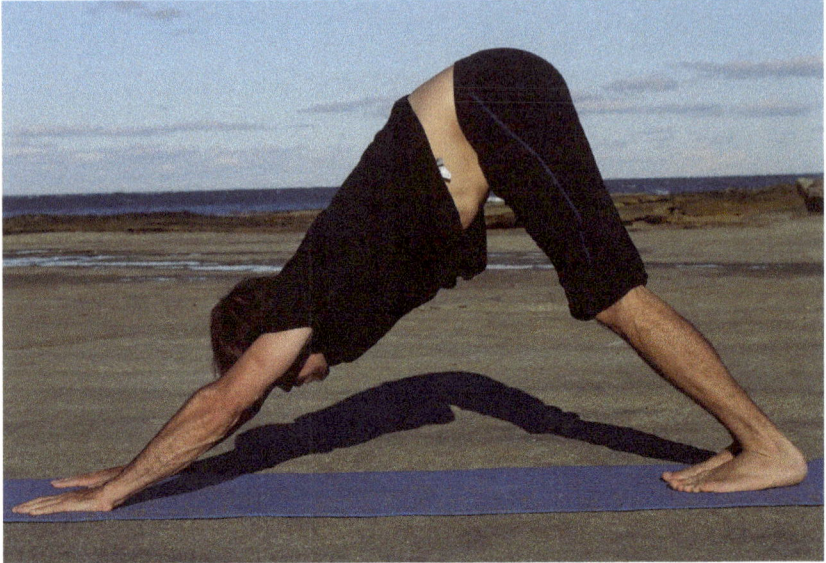

After dog pose you can come into various postures by dropping to the knees and sitting on your heels.

A restful pose is the pose of the child - BALASANA. A meditative pose is diamond posture, known also as the thunderbolt pose, or in Sanskrit VAJRASANA.

## DIAMOND POSTURE - VAJRASANA

Sit up on the heels, spine and head erect. If your body allows, sit on the inner edge of the upturned feet. The fronts of your feet and toes should be flat on the floor.

Have the arms down by your sides, knees and thighs together. The buttocks, or better still, the outer edge of the buttocks will be resting on top of the heels.

*Variation:*

Rest the hands on the thighs. Breathe freely for at least 30 seconds. For meditation in this posture, you might practise a mudra, using the fingers and thumbs such as the GYAN MUDRA: index finger and thumb joined, making a circle.

From VAJRASANA to child posture is an easy transition and vice-versa.

## POSE OF THE CHILD - BALASANA

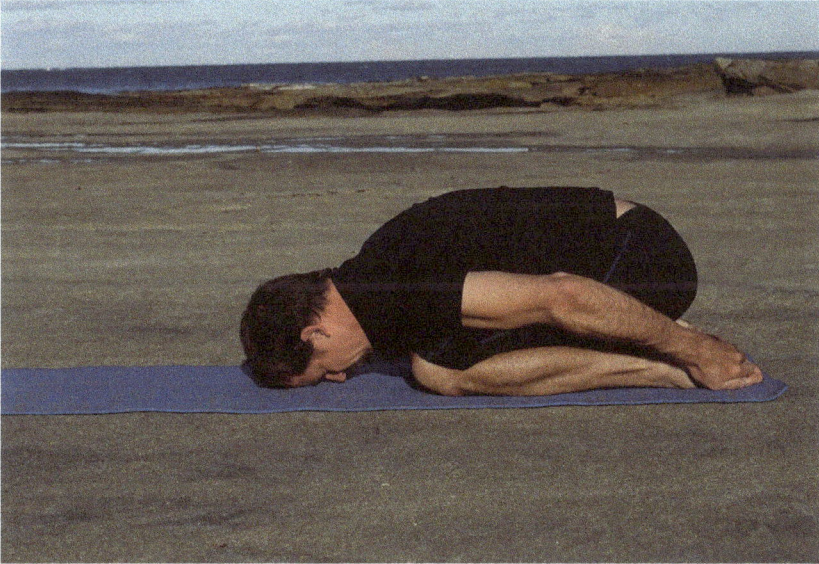

Sitting on your heels with the thighs and knees together, inhale, then on the exhalation simply bend forward and lower the forehead to the floor in front of your knees.

Have your arms by your sides with the backs of your hands on the floor or hold the arches of the feet. The knees can be widened, and big toes joined to give more stretch through the hips.

This wide-legged variation is suggested (with discretion) during pregnancy and for those with a more rounded belly. A cushion for the forehead can also be used.

### CHILD POSE VARIATION - SALAAM POSTURE

Sitting on the heels again, inhale and as you exhale, slide your arms forward together with the head, shoulders and chest, towards the mat.

Have the arms straight. Place the palms of the hands on the floor and lower the forehead to rest on the mat. Aim to keep the buttocks down to the heels.

*Variation:*

Widen the knees to the edge of the mat, keeping the buttocks down between the heels, or on the heels, depending on your body flexibility. Keep your big toes together to form an energy circuit. Stretch out the arms to the floor.

For a more intense back stretch, lift the head so that the face is parallel to the mat and floor, not on it, and not dropped down or poking up. Have your straight arms elevated from the mat; only the palms will be down. Keep the ears in line with your upper arms. Think of the vertebrae of your neck being in line with those of your upper back. Stretch your arms on the mat to elongate the back.

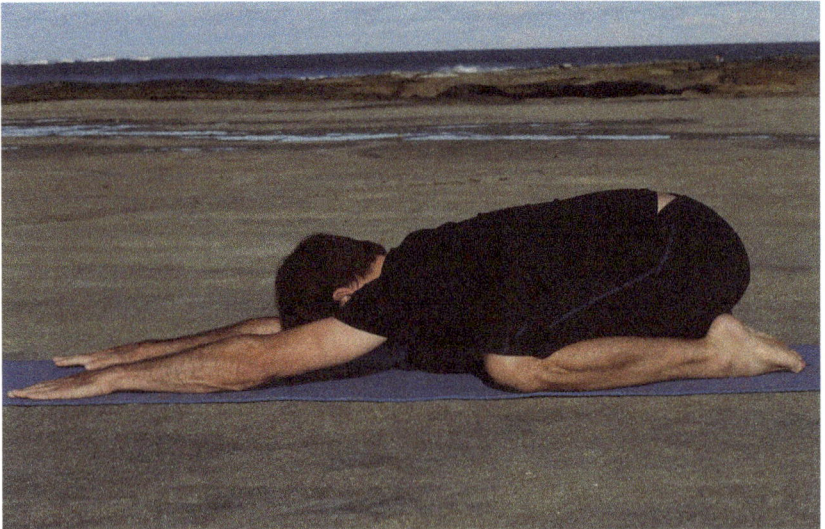

Maintain this longways stretch for at least ten seconds, breathing freely. Next, widen across the shoulders moving the elbows and the outside edge of the armpits slightly outwards, until you can feel a stretch across your back - between the shoulder blades. Finally, bring the hands, one on top of the other under your forehead and rest the head.

## BACK EXERCISE - LOOSENING UP

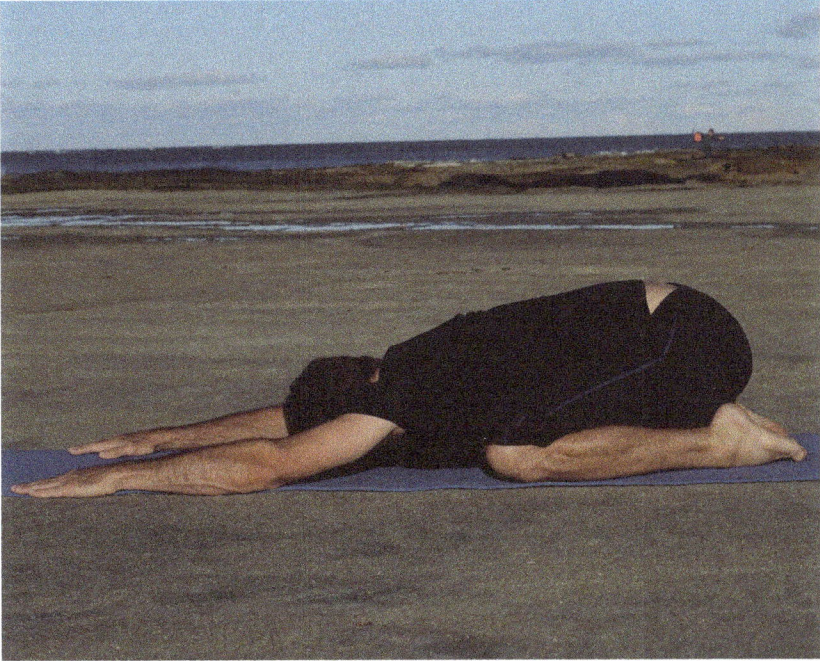

## HINGING BACK AND FORWARD

Bring the knees back together and sit up on your heels in diamond/thunderbolt posture. Breathe in and stretch your arms above your head then as you breathe out, lean forward and take the arms to the mat in front of you, palms down.

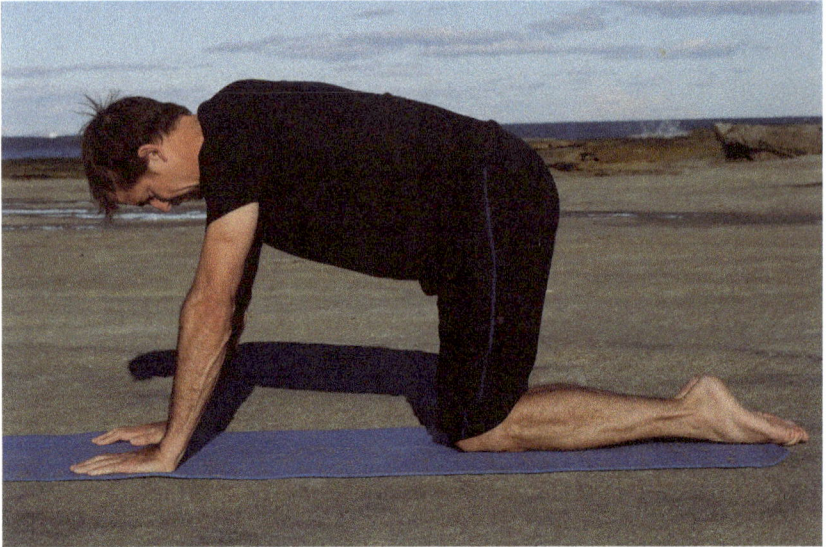

Keeping your hands in the same place, breathe in and come up on the hands and knees. You can also tighten the abdominals as you pause.

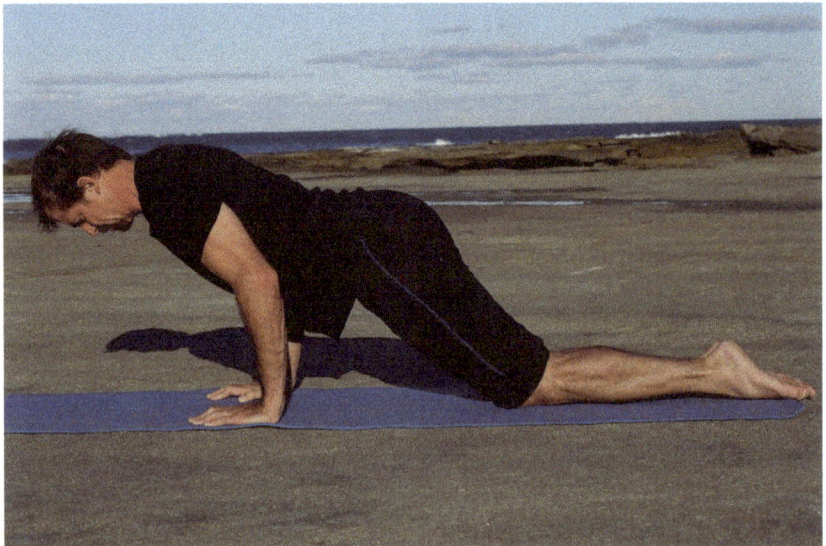

Breathe out and go forward, if possible, without moving the hands or feet.

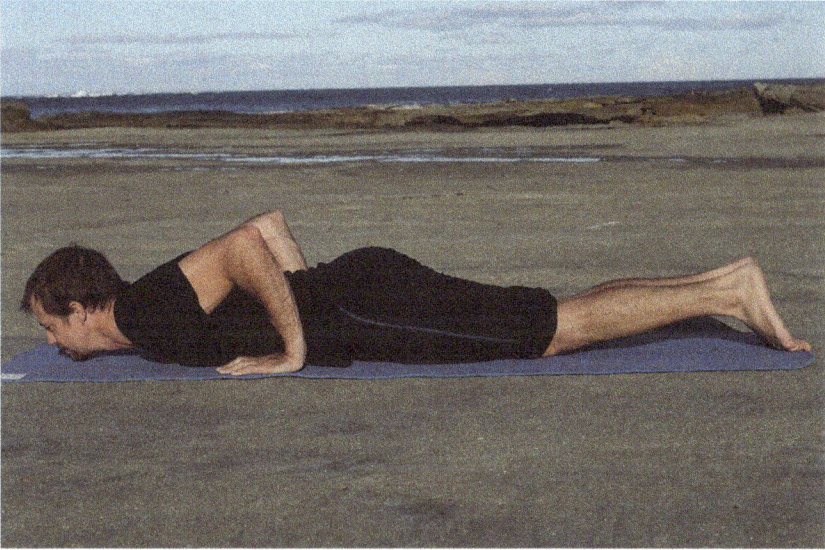

Try and keep the fronts of your feet down on the mat. You will bring your whole body down to the mat. Next, breathe in and come up on the knees.

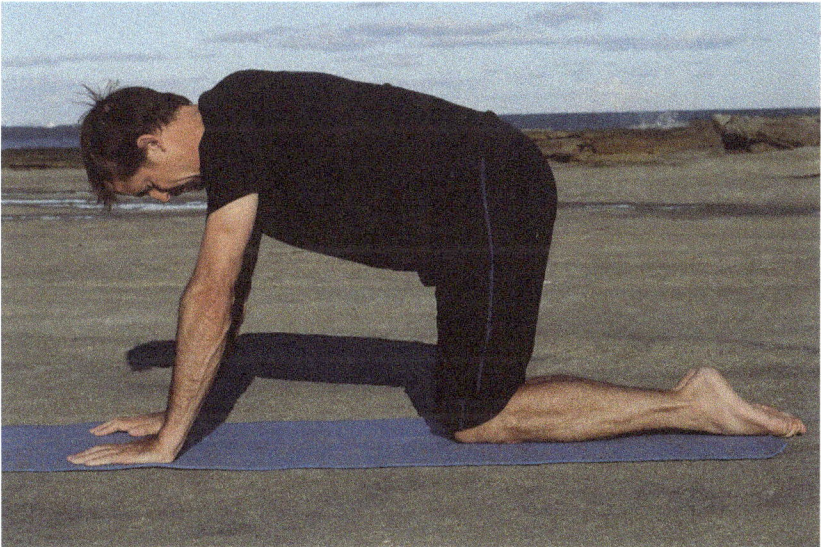

Breathe out, sit down on your heels.

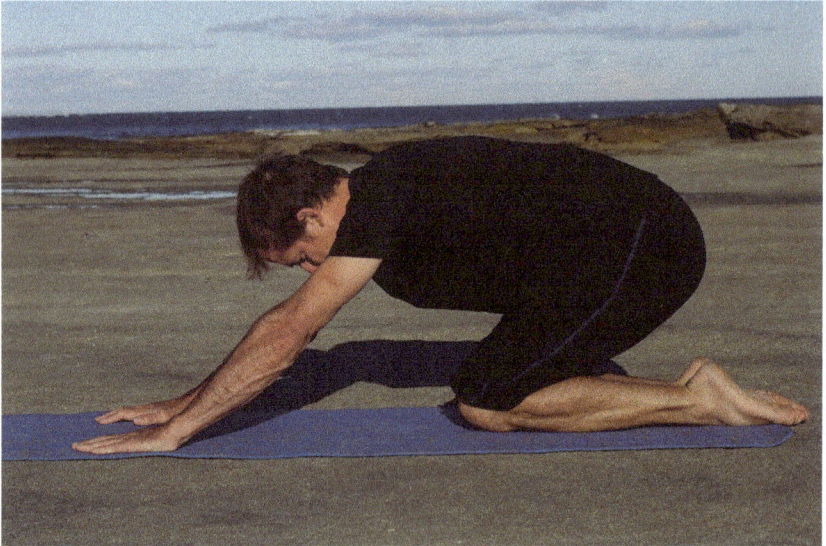

Breathe in - up on the knees, breathe out - hinge forward. Keep doing this for a minute, back and forth with the breath.

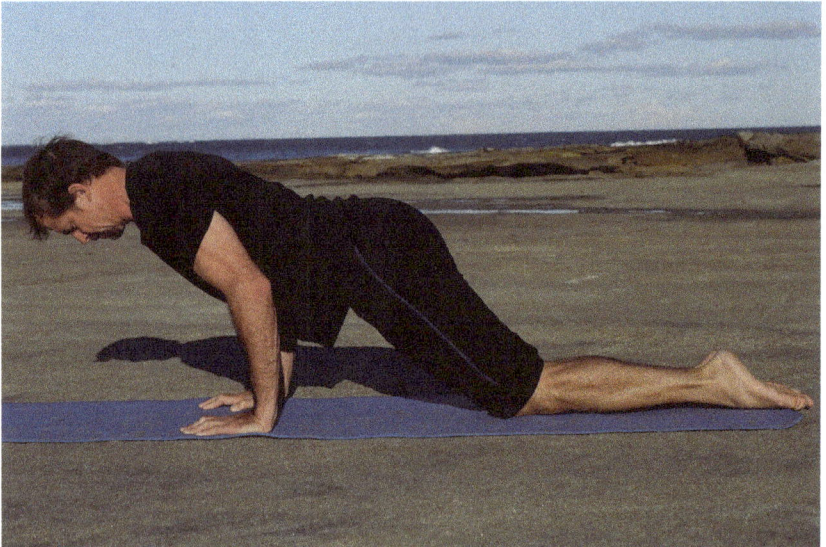

Finally sit back on the heels.

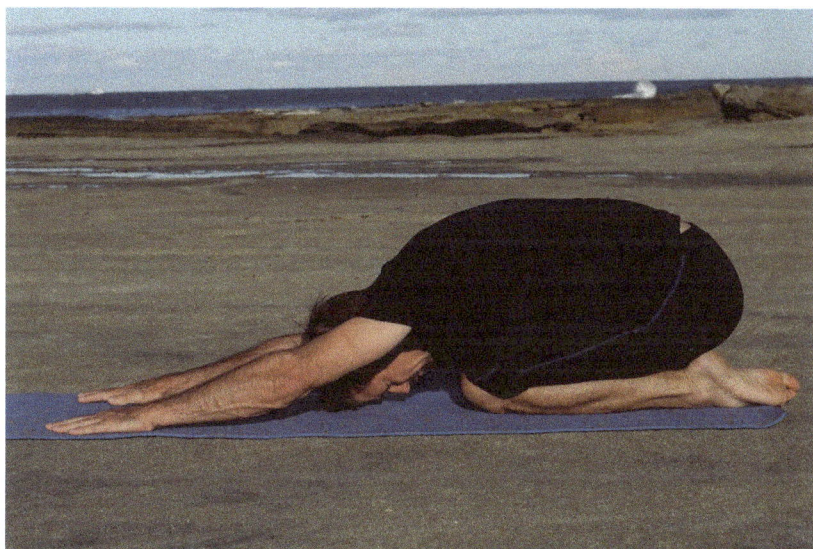

From this posture, either sit up on your heels then use your hands to come into a standing posture, or, assume the cat pose, walk the hands one hand forward, and push up into a dog stretch. Other ways to begin dog stretch will be discussed later in the book.

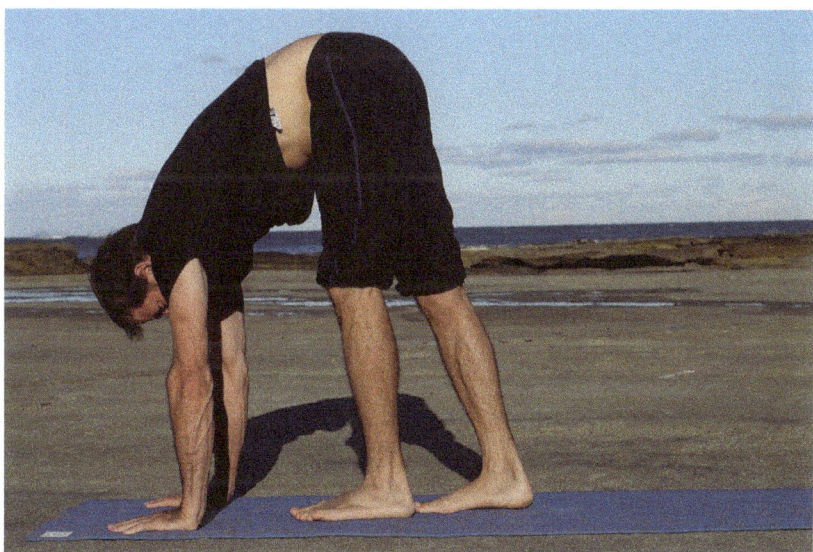

From dog, walk your feet towards your hands, and, vertebra by vertebra, slowly come up into a standing position.

Before we commence some standing asanas, here is an exercise to limber the muscles around the shoulder blades: breathe in, take your right arm up towards your right ear, hold the breath as you bring the arm down to shoulder level, and breathe out as you bring it down close by your side with the wrist very slightly behind the right hip. Do the same with the left arm.

Now roll the shoulders up to your ears, back and down again.

You are ready for some standing stretches. TADASANA, the following pose is the main stance before most standing yoga postures.

# STANDING CORRECTLY AND SALUTE TO THE SUN

## MOUNTAIN POSE - TADASANA

Stand straight with your feet together or as near as is comfortable. Have them in line with each other. Lift the toes and re-seat them, spreading the balls of the feet and distributing weight evenly through the feet.

Have your arms by your sides. Lift the kneecaps and be aware of your thighs. Lift the crown towards the sky and straighten the spine from the crown to the tailbone. Tighten the stomach muscles, engaging the core, and squeeze the shoulder blades towards each other, thus opening the chest.

Check you are standing up straight, feet almost together with the weight distributed evenly, arms by the sides. The head, neck and spine, and the pelvis and legs, are straight. Your hands, side of your hips, knees and ankles will be in line. Check your alignment.

Inhale, take your arms up above your head either side of the ears. Exhale, lower your hands down by your sides ready for SURYA NAMASKAR.

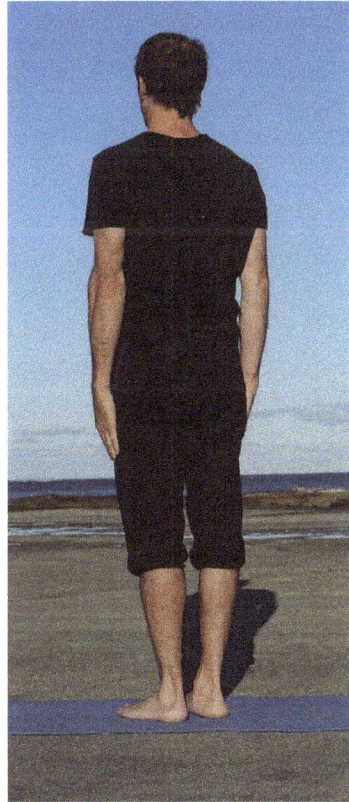

## SALUTE TO THE SUN - SURYA NAMASKAR

For students who have a regular practice, salute to the sun - SURYA NAMASKAR, is a warm up.

However, doing some of the former stretches and postures beforehand will make it easier to do.

Salute to the sun welcomes and reveres the sun. Namaskar means to salute, revere or honour. Coupled with SURYA - the sun, SURYA NAMASKAR means a ritual to worship the sun.

The sun is the source of all forms of life and has long been revered by various cultures for its life-giving properties and as a manifestation of a greater power or divinity.

Salute to the sun, traditionally, should be done in the morning, preferably at sunrise, outside or near an open window. Performing this series of asanas in the morning can help energise the solar plexus - your sun centre.

The sun connects with and energises the solar plexus, which is a centre made up of an intricate web of nerves behind the navel. It gives vitality to both the body and mind. The solar plexus is so called because, like the sun, it radiates and is a source of energy and heat. It corresponds to the energy centre MANIPURA CHAKRA.

In Vedic astrology, the traditional 12 postures of salute to the sun correspond to the 12 signs of the zodiac and their ruling planets. Each pose also has a Sanskrit mantra.

Salute to the sun can assist in the correction of some scoliosis, dowagers hump, arthritis and more. You will begin in the prayer pose.

The postures can be practised as stand-alone asanas or as part of the whole series SURYA NAMASKAR.

## PRAYER POSE - PRANAMASANA

Salute to the sun begins in prayer pose - PRANAMASANA. This pose is for focusing the mind and being still. Be aware of the body as you breathe in and out through the nose.

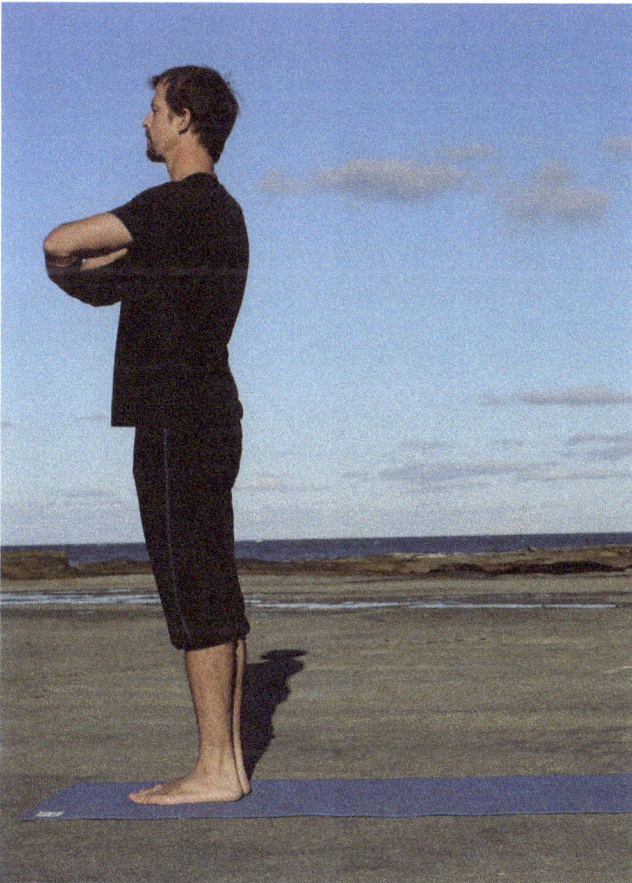

Each 'round' of salute to the sun has two sides. We will work firstly with the right side.

When we come back into the prayer position at the end of *half a round*, we will begin on the left side.

Stand with your palms pressed together in the prayer position, fingers pointing upwards and thumbs towards the breastbone. This is a hand mudra known as ANJALI MUDRA, a salutation seal. Mudra means to seal, and ANJALI to offer, hence: prayer pose.

## UPWARD SALUTE - URDHVA HASTASANA

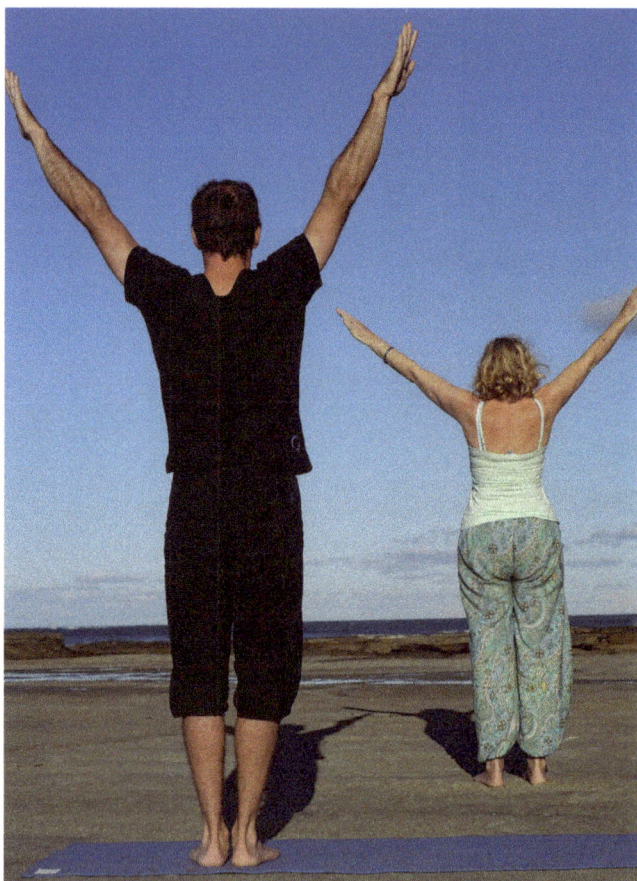

Now take the finger-tips towards the breastbone, so that the heels of the hands are angled away from the body.

Breathe in and stretch your arms slowly upwards above your head, in line with the body, or slightly wider, opening the heart centre. The palms should be open and face forward, fingers-tips stretching out.

Tuck the coccyx in and push the pelvis slightly forward, arching back.

This movement improves posture, relieves tension from the spine and keeps the cartilage between vertebrae in good condition. It opens the chest and in an esoteric sense, the heart centre, symbolising open-heartedness.

Breathe out and stretch forward with a long back, folding forward from the hips into the next posture.

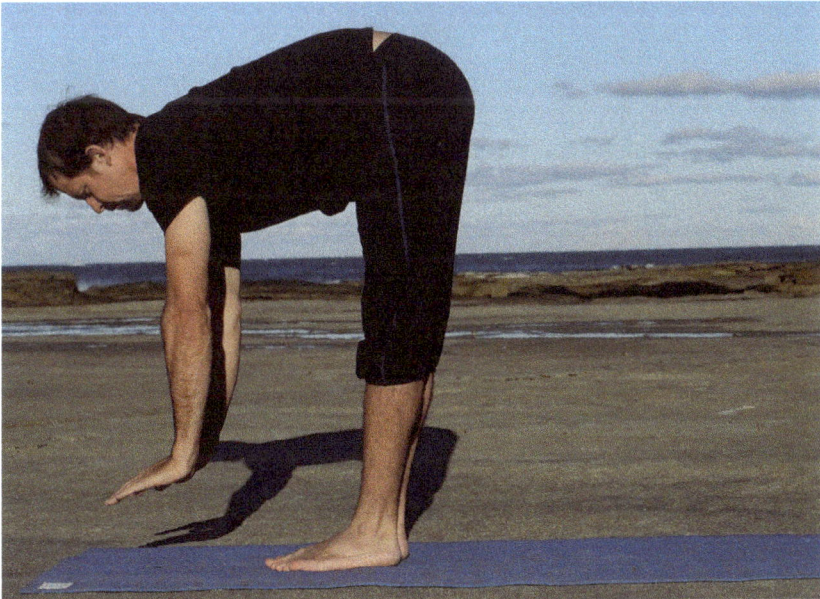

## HEAD TO KNEE - UTTANASANA/PADAHASTASANA

PADAHASTANA means foot and hand posture.

The main difference between this and UTTANASANA is that PADAHASTANA takes the palms under the feet, so that the fingers and palms slide under the toes and balls of the feet. Some traditions have hands fully to the floor, palms down by the sides of the feet, in line with the toes, or to the back of the heels.

UTTANASANA takes the hands to the floor, shins, thighs or wherever they can reach. You can also take the hands behind the legs to hold the heels. This is also a 'hands to feet pose', you could say!

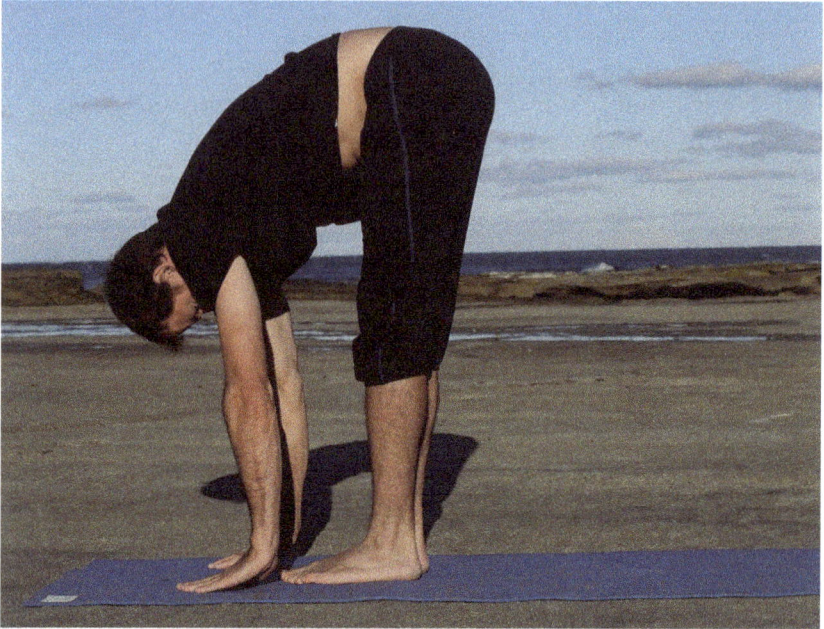

To continue: As you exhale, take your hands to the ground in line with your feet and take your abdomen to your thighs, followed by the chest.

Rest the head against or beyond the knees. Keep the legs straight. Initially you may need to soften the knees to accommodate the body lowering to the thighs.

If you have high or low blood pressure, place the hands on the shins and come half-way into a table top. From there, lift the upper chest to be very slightly higher than the hips, keeping the head neutral or slightly up.

Traditional SURYA NAMASKAR takes the body down with the chest to the thighs and head towards the knees. This is a good massage for the digestive system.

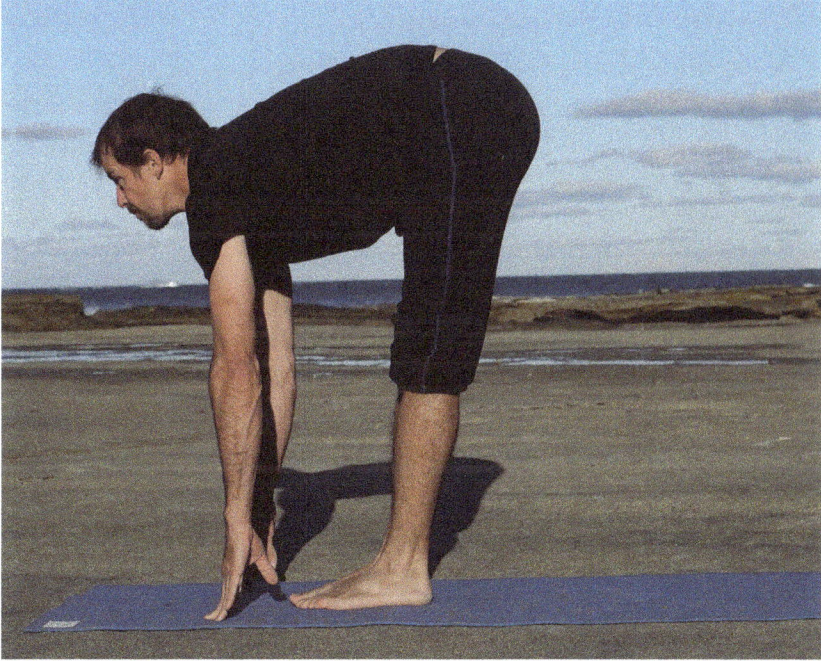

Some variations of UTTANASANA, particularly as a 'stand-alone' posture, after taking the head to the knees, come half way up to engage and stretch the long muscles of the back.

This becomes ARDHA UTTANASANA - the half forward fold. If using the half forward fold, slowly straighten the legs and rest the hands on the shins.

From head to knee posture, or as near as possible, keeping a long back, place the hands on the mat down by the feet.

In salute to the sun, the next posture is the equestrian pose and it is a lunge back. As this is the first side of SURYA NAMASKAR, you will lunge back with the right leg.

### THE EQUESTRIAN (LUNGES) - ASHWA SANCHALANASANA

The posture is good for the hip, knee and ankle joints.

Lift the head up, inhale and lunge back with your right leg. Drop the right/back knee to the mat, toes gripping the mat. Have the left/ front knee, initially, in line with the ankle, foot between the hands.

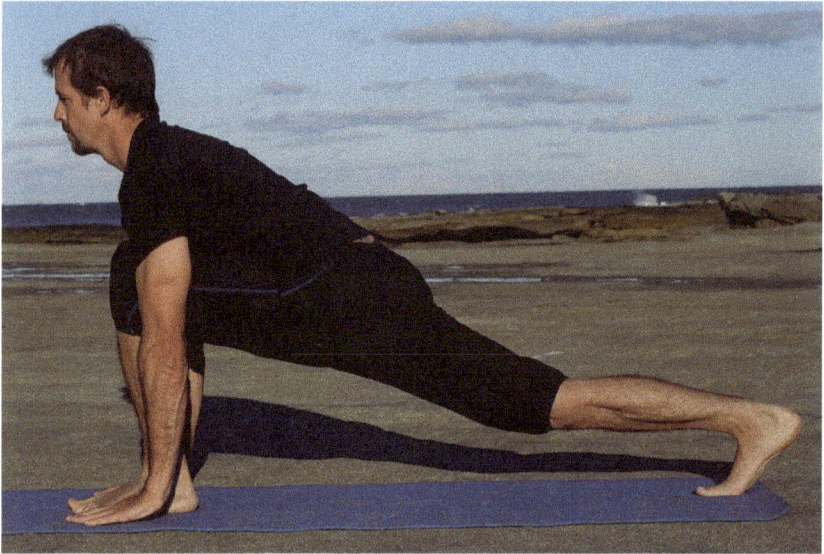

For an additional, extra stretch, if your knees and ankles are strong, you can take your left knee forward, beyond the ankle, to hide your big toe.

It provides a good stretch, creating space between joints. Should your knees or ankles not accommodate this extra stretch, simply maintain alignment of keeping the knee over the ankle. Either way, retain the breath and lift the right knee.

Traditionally, the breath is held from here through to the next pose, breathing out for the pose of forehead, chin, chest after the plank, but it might be suggested that you initially breathe as needed. With practice, retain the inhalation as you move into the following posture: KUMBHAKASANA.

## THE PLANK/WHEELBARROW - KUMBHAKASANA

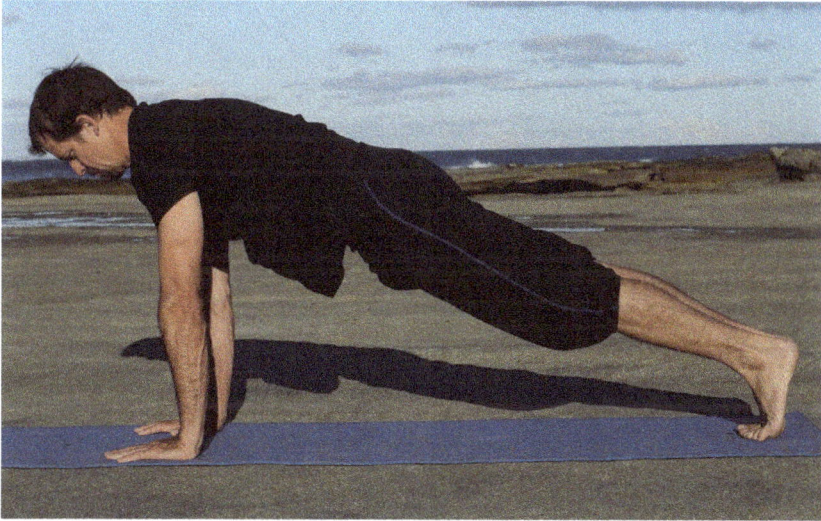

Press the back toes into the mat. After lifting the right knee, straighten the right leg.

Take the left leg back alongside the right. Now your body should be in a line from the head to the heels. This is the plank posture - also named the wheelbarrow. You will be supporting yourself on your hands and toes.

KUMBHAKA comes from the Sanskrit word KUMBHAK, which means breath retention. You inhale on the lunge back with the right leg, hold the breath through the rest of the equestrian pose, through the plank, and exhale on the next pose - the forehead, chin and chest pose which resembles a caterpillar or earthworm. Obviously, if you decide to hold the plank posture for strength - just breathe normally!

Only hold the breath if you are moving through salute to the sun without lengthy posture holds. Even then, you might elect to breathe out when the knee lunges forward, (before the plank) and inhale before the plank and still hold the breath until the forehead chest-chin pose - it's just that you managed to get an extra breath in.

This posture tones the nervous centres along the spine. It also tones the stomach muscles and strengthens the back, neck, shoulders, arms and legs.

## KNEES-CHEST-CHIN POSE - ASHTANGA NAMASKARA

From plank, exhale, dropping to the knees.

Bend the arms and lower the upper chest, the forehead and/or chin. Your hands shouldn't move, and the finger-tips will be roughly in line with your shoulders. The elbows are kept high.

Press the chin down towards the hollow beneath it and slide the forehead through between the hands. At the same time, keep the base of the spine angled upwards, towards the sky.

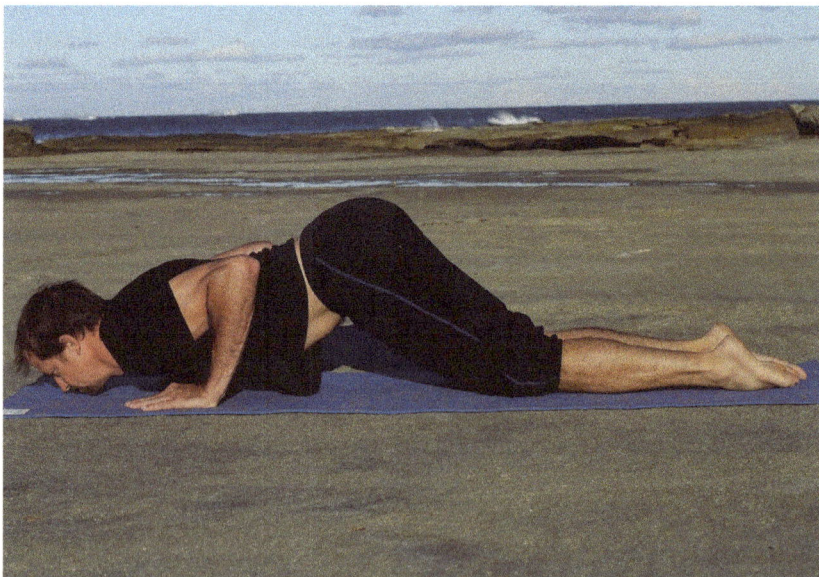

Keeping the pelvis and coccyx (rear end) up, abdominal muscles in, have your toes curled under until you lower the hips. Then point the toes away.

Keep the shoulder blades pushed together to avoid shoulder injury. Think of how flexible an earthworm or caterpillar is and how they move along the ground.

Fully lower your body.

## THE COBRA - BHUNGANASANA

From having lowered the body to the mat, the fingertips should still be in line with shoulders.

Breathe in and raise the head, neck and chest into the cobra pose. Look up. The spine should be slowly bent back until you are able to straighten the arms or as near as possible. Both versions are shown.

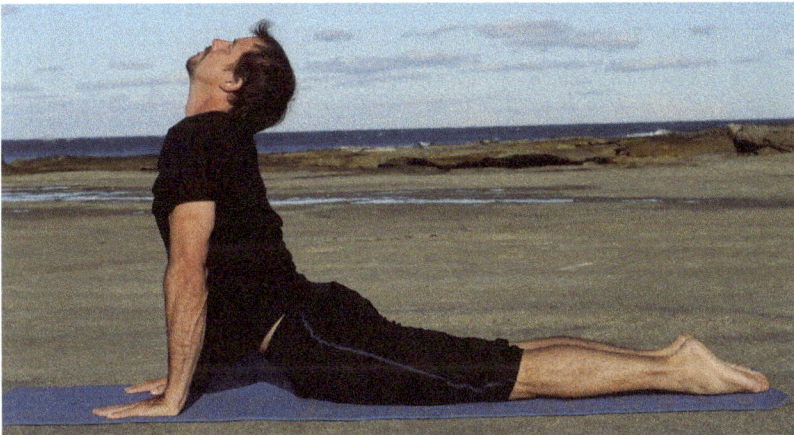

You will be supporting the body with the legs, pelvis and hands. Keep the thighs on the ground. If you can, keep the pelvis also on the ground.

Relax the shoulders. The pressure on your middle back is where the adrenal glands are receiving a good massage. The cobra and the knees-chest-chin pose are good postures for anxiety, depression and stress. The cobra also exercises the spine and stretches the chest.

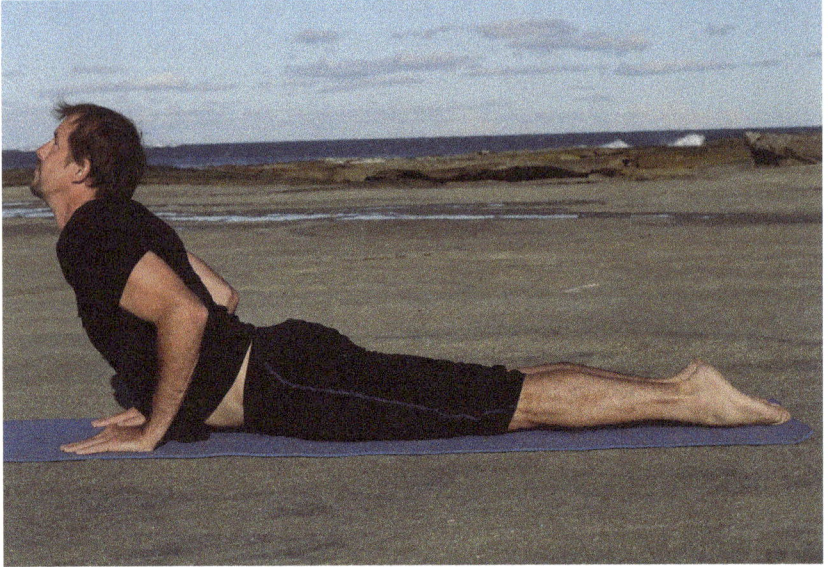

If you are performing BHUNGANASANA as an isolated pose, and not after sliding through with ASHTANGA NAMASKARA as part of SURYA NAMASKAR, you will begin with your body on the floor, face downwards, chin on the ground and fingertips in line with your shoulders.

Breathe in, lifting the head, chest and shoulders from the floor. Ideally the arms will be straight but take care not to hunch the shoulders. It's better that the arms bend slightly and that the shoulders are relaxed. Push up until the upper body is stretching up and bend back from the waist. Bend the spine as much as you are able. Relax the buttocks and shoulders; let the head drop back. Hold for several seconds. Breathing out, slowly lower the body down and relax, arms by your sides, head to one side. The cobra strengthens the spine, spinal nerves and back muscles.

From the cobra, breathe out and push the hips up.

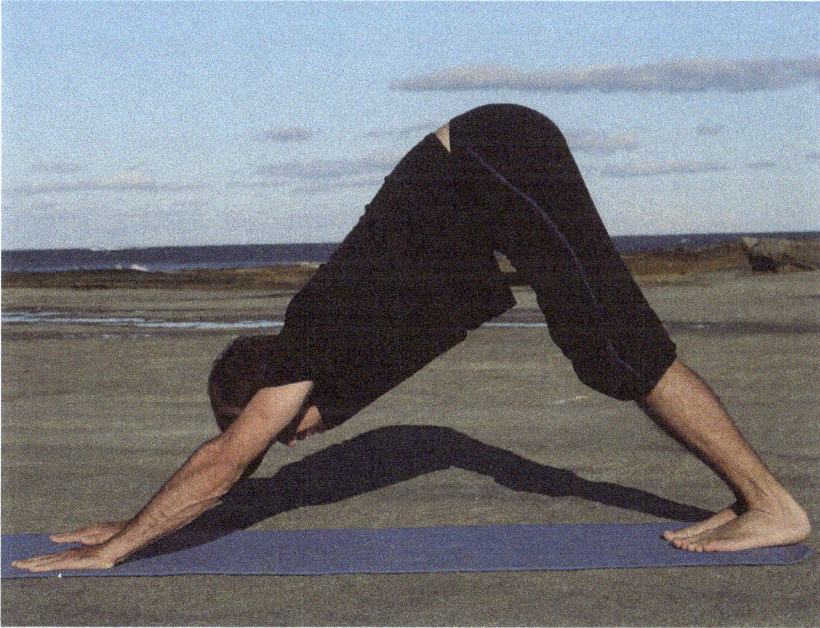

## ADHO MUKHA SVANASANA - DOG STRETCH

As you thrust up the hips, elevate the coccyx so that the body forms an upside-down 'V' shape then swing the head through between the arms.

Ease the heels to the ground if you are able. Aim to flatten and straighten the back all the way to the shoulders.

Pull the abdomen in towards the spine.

Dog stretch is good for the whole back and muscles in the back, shoulders and legs.

Breathe in, lunge your right leg through between your hands and bring your chest forward into the equestrian pose.

## THE EQUESTRIAN (LUNGES)
## - ASHWA SANCHALANASANA again.

The right knee lunges forward. Drop the back/left knee.

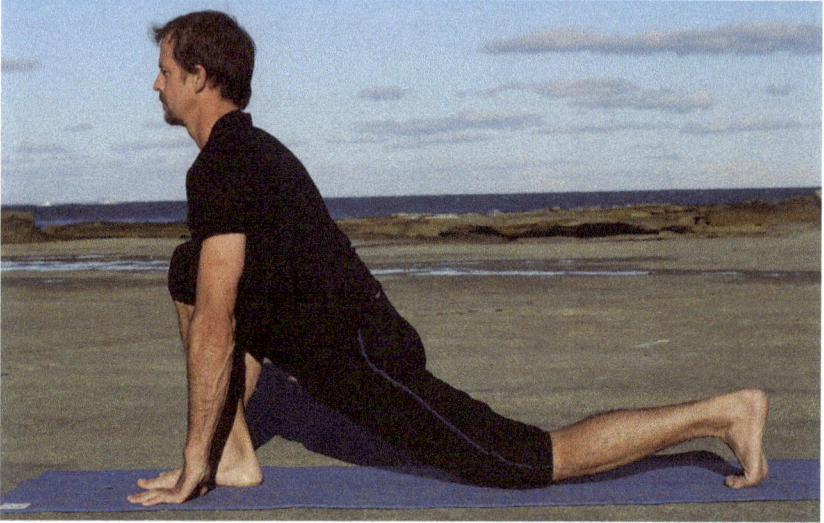

Lift the knee and step the leg through to the front of the mat lifting your hips.

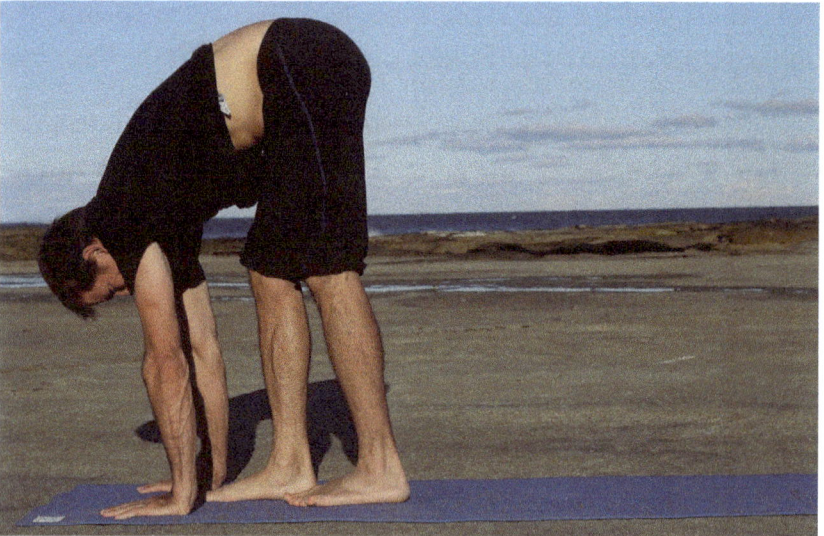

Breathe out, bring the head to the knees, hands wrapped around your ankles or grasp your heels, in **UTTANASANA**, the head to knee posture. Alternatively place them flat down by the sides of your feet or under the feet in **PADAHASTANA**.

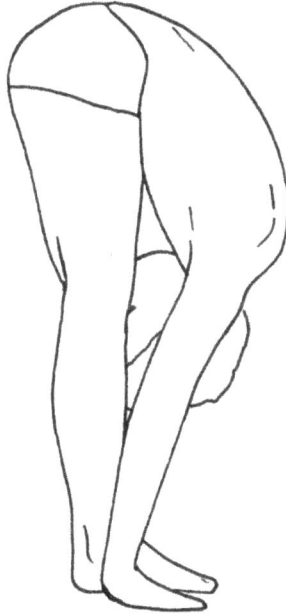

In the full head-to-knee pose the digestive system receives a massage. If this is uncomfortable, come into ARDHA UTTANASANA bringing the hands to the shins and lifting the upper chest slightly higher than the hips.

From head-to-knee or the half-way option, breathe in and take your hands and arms up above your head in the upward salute - URDHVA HASTASANA, as if greeting the morning sun, as we began.

Breathing out, bring the hands into prayer position, PRANAMASANA, then take them down via the face and chest to the breastbone, thumbs interlaced. YOU HAVE NOW COMPLETED **HALF A ROUND** OF SALUTE TO THE SUN.

<u>**Start again**</u>, **for the second side**.

### PRAYER POSE - PRANAMASANA

Bring the hands into prayer pose. This time you'll be lunging with the opposite leg.

### UPWARD SALUTE - URDHVA HASTASANA

Inhale. Stretch the arms up above the head, opening the upper chest and tilting the pelvis forward slightly. Next, exhale, into forward bend, head to knee.

### HEAD TO KNEE - UTTANASANA / PADAHASTASANA

From head to knee, breathe in and lunge back with the left leg this time.

### THE EQUESTRIAN (LUNGES)
### - ASHWA SANCHALANASANA

Allow the front/left knee to soften forward when you drop the back/right knee - if the knees and ankles are strong.

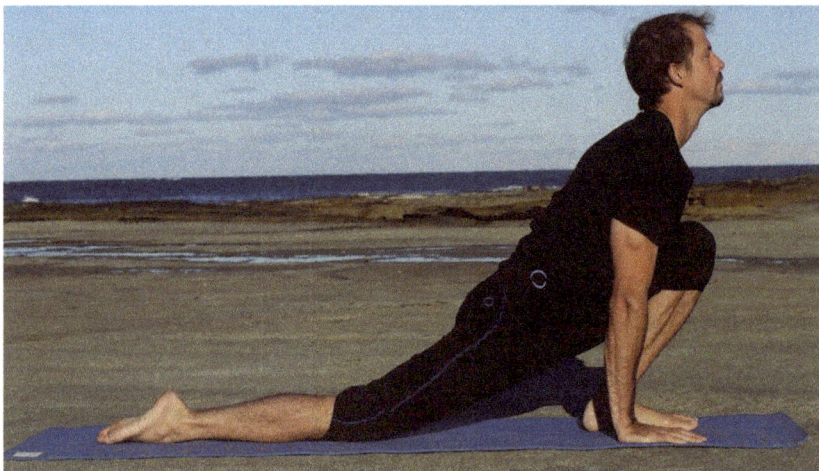

Drop the back knee to the floor. Ideally, hold the breath through to the next pose which will be the plank.
Take the front leg back in line with the back leg so that your body is in a line from the neck to the heel.

## THE PLANK/WHEELBARROW - KUMBHAKASANA

Hold the breath through the plank, if comfortable. You'll breathe out during the next posture.

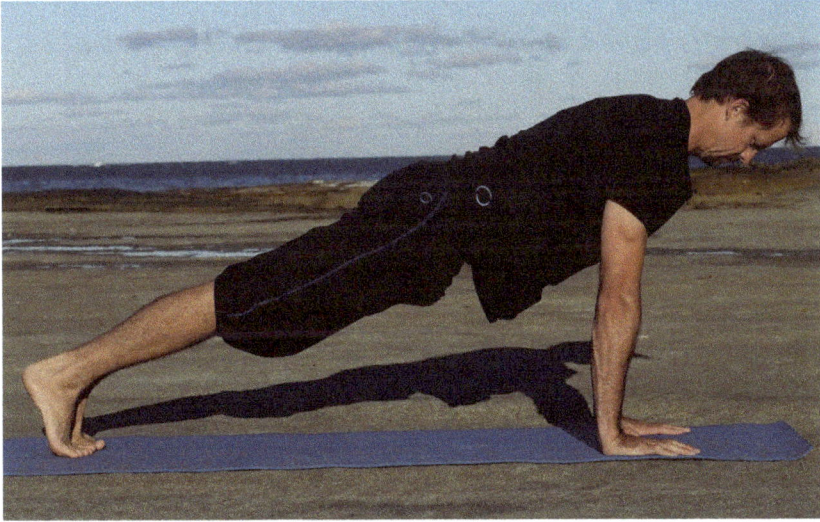

Tighten the abdominals (except during pregnancy), drop to the knees, bend the elbows and take the chest and forehead between the hands, breathing out.

## KNEES-CHEST-CHIN POSE - ASHTANGA NAMASKARA

Slither through into knees-chest-chin pose, keeping the pelvis up. (See following page).

From there, when the whole body is finally down on the mat, breathe in and push up into:

## COBRA - BHUNGASANA

Arch back. Aim to straighten the arms.

# YOGA - KEEPING IT UP

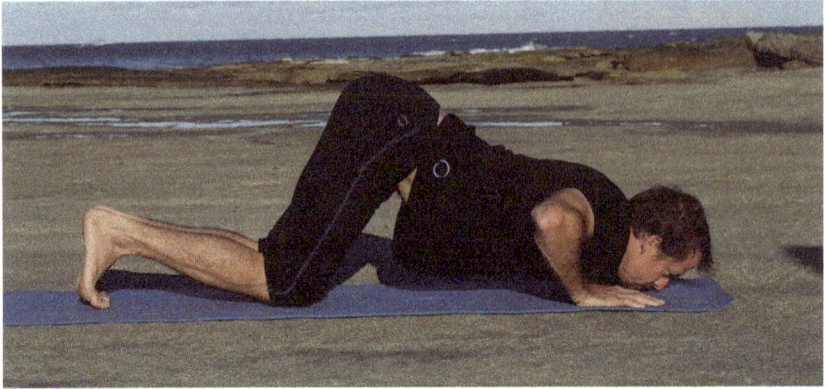

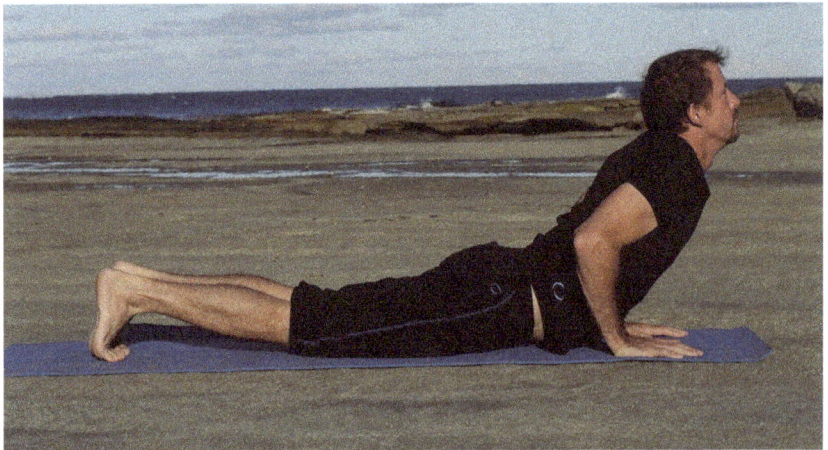

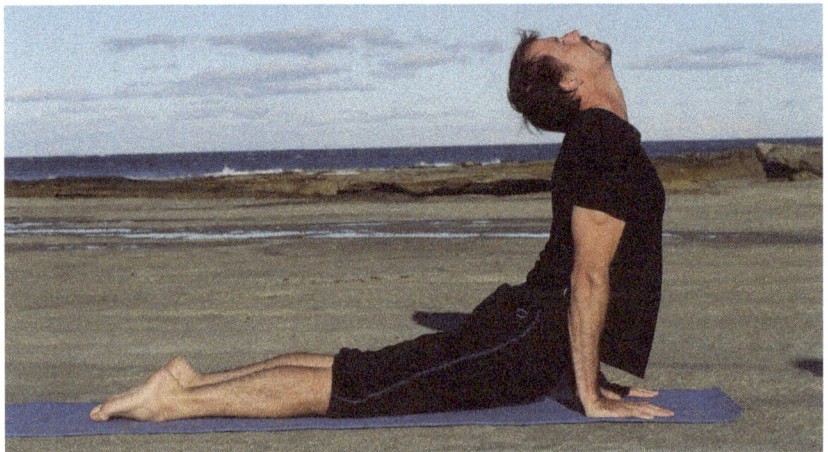

## DOG STRETCH - ADHO MUKHA SVANASANA

From cobra, soften the back, tuck the toes in, exhale and raise the hips. Straighten the legs, heels to the mat if you are able. Bring the coccyx up. Swing the head and trunk down between your straight arms. Press down with the heels of the hands. Hands and feet equal distance apart.

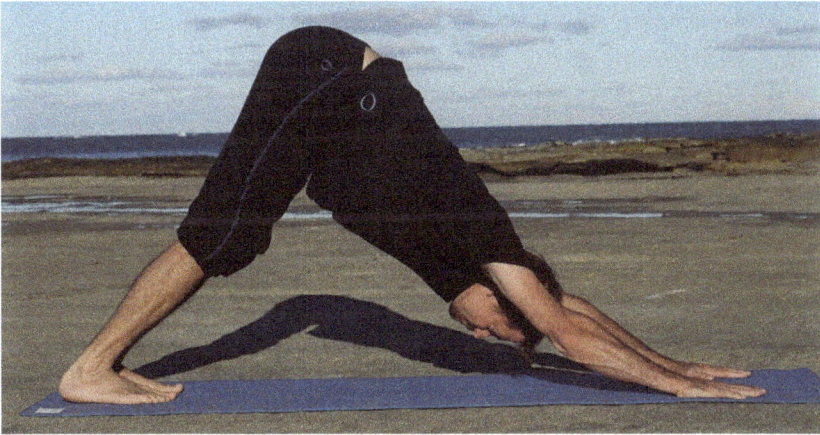

If approaching the dog stretch as an isolated posture rather than as part of the series salute to the sun, begin in a cat position with the hands under the shoulders and the knees under the hips. Simply walk the hands one hand measurement forward, then push up the hips so that your body is like an upside-down 'V' shape. Also, you can begin in a standing position, with the whole yoga mat in front of you. Breathe in and stretch the arms up, breathe out, stretch forward from the hips and lower your hands to the space in front of your feet. Feel free to soften your knees. With the palms fully on the mat, walk forward until your heels just begin to lift on the floor, then remain in that position with the hips up and the hands and feet on the ground.

### THE EQUESTRIAN (LUNGES) - ASHWA SANCHALANASANA

Continuing salute to the sun from the dog stretch: Breathe in and lunge forward with the left foot, into the equestrian.

Lower your right/back knee to the mat, then lift the right/back knee and step the right foot forward between the arms.

Exhale as you straighten both legs into:

### PADAHASTANA or UTTANASANA

Lift the coccyx towards the sky and take your head to your knees (as far as you comfortably are able). Now wrap your hands around your ankles in the head to knee posture.

Breathe in, bring your arms up either side of your ears, into:

### UPWARD SALUTE - URDHVA HASTASANA

and come into a standing position.

### PRANAMASANA

Breathe out and lower your hands into the prayer position, passing by the face to the chest and the heart centre. Still the mind.

This completes one whole round of salute to the sun, starting with the right side, and secondly with the left.

> Approaching **UTTANASANA** as a stand-alone posture, begin from a standing position. Have the feet shoulder width apart and ground them into the mat. Breathe in and as you breathe out bend from the waist and stretch the back out then lower it, together with the arms towards your ankles, taking the chest and stomach to the thighs and the head towards the knees. Wrap the hands around the ankles.

Three rounds of salute to the sun in the morning will help keep the body healthy and flexible.

If you wish to simply do a couple of lunges, left and right, exhale and push up into dog pose, after the pose of the child and the cat-cow pose. Breathe in and lunge first with your right leg, bringing the foot between the hands, and dropping the left knee. Lift the head. Step back into dog pose exhaling. Next time, breathe in and lunge forward with the left foot, bringing the foot between the hands, lift the head and drop the right knee. Exhale and this time bring the right foot forward and straighten both legs. Fold from the hips towards the knees. Lift the coccyx towards the sky. Take your chest forward towards your thighs. Finally take the head to the knees. Breathe in and either stretch up, arms above your head, or gently roll the spine up vertebra by vertebra.

# SECTION 3

## STANDING STRETCHES

### GENTLE TRIANGLE

Stand on the mat with the feet at least one metre apart. Raise one arm and stretch to the opposite toes, or ankles, then do the same with the other side. Keep stretching your right hand to your left ankle and your left hand to your right ankle alternatively.

Breathe in as you come up, breathe out to an ankle. Finally, hold a right or left ankle with the opposite hand, stretching across your body and maintain for a few seconds. As you do so, raise the other arm up and look towards the palm. Now do the same with the opposite hand and foot.

This **triangle** posture is a good warm up for stronger versions and can generally be practised by those with lower back pain without difficulty.

### THE AXE BREATH

From the gentle triangle pose, bring both hands to the mat between your feet, and bend and stretch the legs, trying to keep your hands on the ground as you straighten the legs.

While breathing exercises are done in a sitting posture, traditionally, this is nevertheless a good place to practise a few 'HA' breaths.

The 'HA' or AXE breath is good practice for both UJJYI and KAPALABHATI described towards the end of the book, where you will breathe in *and out* through the nose, making a similar sound to the 'Ha' breath about to be described - breathing out now - through the mouth.

Begin with your legs wide and hands on the mat between each ankle, clasp the hands as if holding an axe. Breathe in through the nose, raise your upper body and stretch your clasped hands over your head.

Come forward from the hips, swinging your clasped hands forward as if chopping wood. At the same time as your body sways forward, breathe out forcefully through the mouth with a 'ha' sound.

This helps expel stale air from the bottom of the lungs. Repeat the breath another two times.

Tuck the chin in, narrow the stance of your feet to about hip width and slowly round up, vertebra by vertebra. When the body is upright raise the chin and roll the shoulders back.

Before the breathing exercise you were introduced to one type of triangle pose.

The following version is a little stronger.

## THE TRIANGLE - TRIKONASANA

Use the *former* option if you find the triangle below uncomfortable, due to a sway back or back pain when holding the posture.

Have your body facing the same way as the LONG edge of your mat. Stand with your legs as wide apart as is comfortable for stability.

Have the right foot only, turned towards the short end or top of the mat. Let's say your body faces north and your foot east.

Have the heel of the front foot in line with the arch of the back foot on an imaginary centre line through the mat.

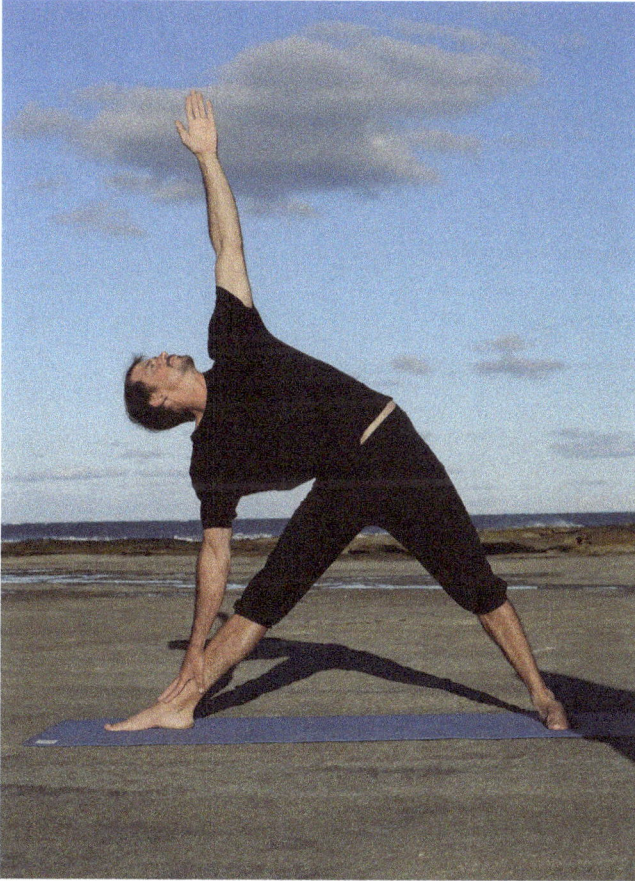

Pivot your left/back foot slightly inwards so the toes angle more towards the long edge of the mat.

Raise your arms up to shoulder level, parallel to the floor and palms facing down. Stretch through the fingertips. Inhale.

As you exhale, reach forward with your right hand in the same direction as your right foot. Allow the body to extend from the hip following the direction of the right hand. Rest your hand on the outer right shin.

If more flexible, place your right fingertips or palm on the floor to the outside of your right shin, behind the leg.

An easier version is to rest your hand on the inside of your calf or ankle. You can also use a block to rest your hand on, as a means of easing nearer to the floor.

As you lower the front hand down towards the calf or ankle, take the back arm (left) up. Keep both shoulders in alignment. Turn your left palm forward, with your fingertips reaching towards the sky.

As you assume the position, ease your left hip back towards the wall behind your left heel. Press down with the little-toe edge of your back/left foot.

Try not to let the upper shoulder bend forward.

Revolve the trunk upwards; gently turn your head and lift the gaze to your left thumb; if stressful for the neck, simply face forward.

Hold for a few seconds and deep breathe, in and out through the nose.

Breathe in and bring the arms up to shoulder level; breathe out and relax the arms.

Change the feet so now the right foot is your back foot, angled slightly forward to the long edge of the mat.

The left foot should face outwards to the short edge of your mat, but your body to the long edge of the mat. Let's say the body faces north and your left foot to the west.

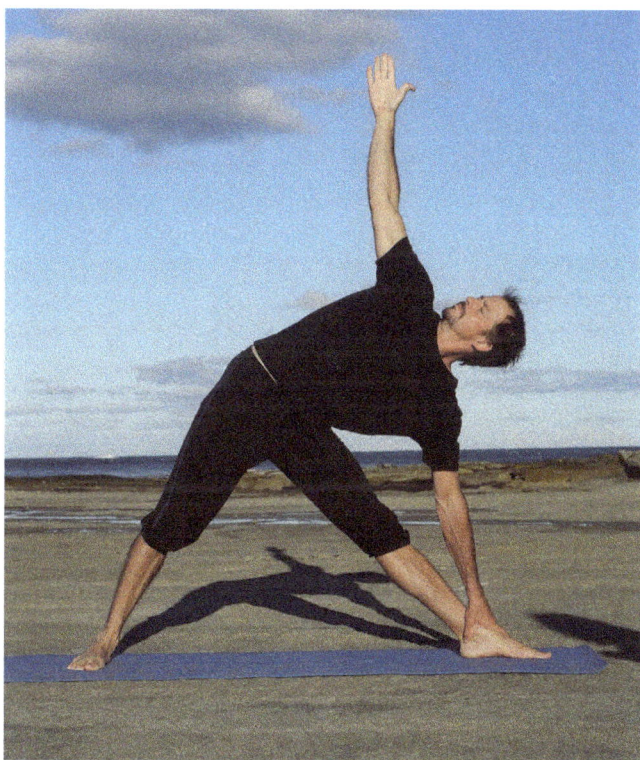

Breathe in and bring the arms up to shoulder level, breathe out and begin stretching towards your left/front calf or ankle. Breathe in and bring the right arm up. Hold for a few seconds. Breathe in and out through the nose.

Finally, breathe in and bring the arms up to shoulder level; breathe out and relax the arms. Bring the feet together and come into TADASANA, mountain pose.

## THE TRIANGLE - TRIKONASANA (AGAINST A WALL)

Now try this posture against a wall, to see how far you're able to stretch with one hand, while keeping the shoulder of the raised hand aligned against the wall.

Take your mat with the long length to the wall. Stand as for the triangle pose described above.

Here, one student has the right foot forward and one has the left foot forward. Breathe in and bring the arms up to shoulder level. As you breathe out, extend your front arm towards your leg. Take the back arm up and gaze towards your thumb.

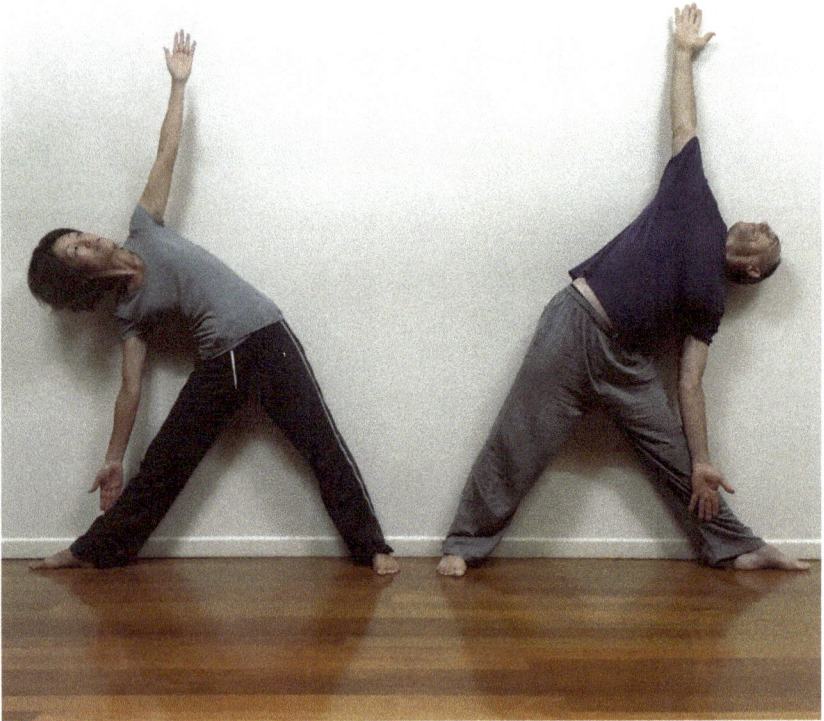

If the shoulder comes forward, ease up slightly. As students become more flexible, over time, the arms and ankle will line up. Breathe in and straighten up, bringing your arms up to shoulder level. Breathe out and release the arms.

The pose stretches the waist and ribs. The hips are stretched and strengthened, as are the knees, thighs and ankles. TRIKONASANA may reduce sciatica. Additionally, the abdominal organs are stimulated, improving digestion.

Maintain a wide-legged stance on your mat, then turn your right foot and your body to face the short edge of the mat ready for:

## THE REVOLVING TRIANGLE POSTURE - PARIVRTTA TRIKONASA

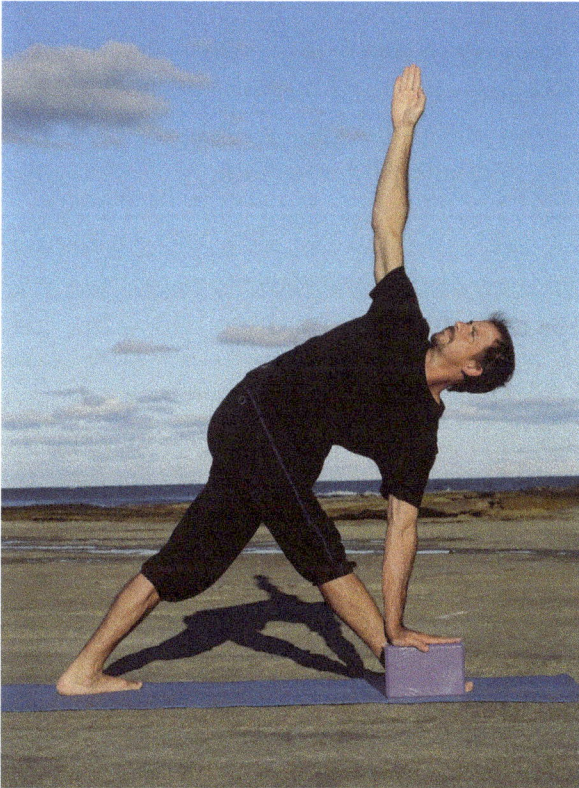

*NOTE: Do not do this pose if you have a slipped disc, burst disc or other vertebral issue.*

Start with the right foot forward and the back/left foot at a slight angle, for stability.

Position a block against the little-toe edge of the right foot.

Draw the left hip and side of the body around in the same direction as your right foot. Ease the right side of your body slightly back, so that the hips are even - both facing the short edge of the mat and your right foot. Try pressing the right thigh back and the left thigh forward.

Bring your hands to your hips to ensure you have squared your hips forward in the same direction as your right foot.

Now breathe in and raise your left arm and extend it forward. Breathe out and hinge forward from your hips stretching your left arm across your body.

Keep your spine long and straight. Place your left hand to the block outside your right foot and open your torso to the right side. Breathe in and raise the right arm to the sky, opening the shoulder, palm forward. Turn your head to gaze towards the right thumb. If you have any neck issues, maintain a neutral head position and look forward into the room or to the space in front of you.

Maintain the posture for a few seconds, increasing to 30 seconds over time, breathing in and out through the nose.

Breathe in and raise the body, arms out, facing forward. Turn to the left long edge of your mat, breathe out and release the arms down.

Repeat on the other side, standing with the left foot pointing towards the short end of the mat. Have the block by the left little-toe edge of the foot. Ease the body around to face the left/front foot, the hips facing the short edge of the mat.

Breathe in and raise your right arm; extend it forward. Breathe out and lean forward from the hips then take your right hand to the readily placed block outside the left ankle. Raise your left arm and look toward the left hand.

Breathe in and come up, face forward to your extended front foot, turn to the right side, breathe out and lower the arms.

The **revolved** triangle pose opens the chest and shoulders and has similar benefits to the triangle. It stretches the groin, hips and spine and strengthens and stretches the legs. This pose also stimulates the abdominal organs, improving digestion, and, it is also good for improving balance.

## HALF MOON - ARDHA CHANDRASANA

Take your mat and place it long-ways up to the wall.

Have the little toe edge of your right foot in line with the wall but a few centimetres away from it, and legs wide as if you are positioned for the triangle pose.

Place a block in front of your foot, about one to one and a half of your foot-lengths away from your toes and in line with them.

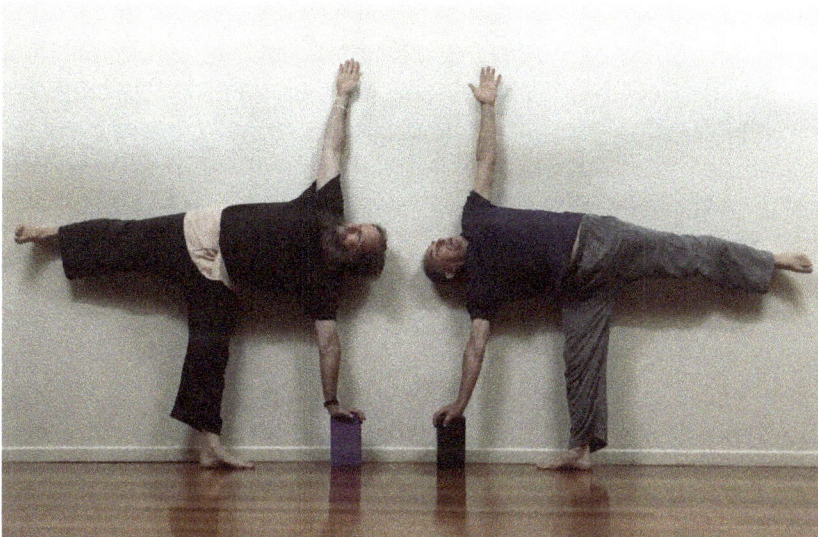

Exhaling, bend your right knee and place your right hand on the block. Raise and stretch the left leg up with the heel towards the wall. Straighten the right knee.

Breathe normally. If you are flexible, or have long limbs,

you will be able to do this posture without a block. In this case place the fingertips on the floor.

Roll the left shoulder and ribs up, and to help you balance, rest the back of the right shoulder lightly against the wall.

Straighten the right arm as you firm the hand into the block, then raise your left arm up in line with it, palm forward.

Rest your left hip and your head against the wall and aim to turn the whole torso upwards towards the wall. Don't let the head drop. For those more accustomed to the pose, roll the back of the head against the wall to look up at the raised hand.

Ease the flesh on the left thigh upwards towards the wall, opening the left hip more.

Depending on shoulder issues, some students, particularly beginners, should place the left hand on the left hip rather than raising it to the wall. Similarly, beginners and those who have any neck problems, don't turn your head to look upward. Simply gaze straight forward with the head in a neutral position and aim to keep both sides of the neck even.

Hold for at least six seconds. Now exhale, bend the right knee, gently lower the left leg, straighten the right one and come into TRIKONASANA.

Now repeat on the other side, turning the left foot to the short edge of the mat with the little toe edge of your left foot centimetres from the wall, your left hand on the block. Exhale, bend the left knee and inhale raise the right leg, shoulder and ribs. Roll the flesh of the thigh towards the wall and open the hip in the same upward direction on this side. Hold for several seconds, free breathing.

Exhale, bend the left knee and lower the right leg. Come into TRIKONASANA.

If you usually practise without wall support, have the block in front of your foot, but a little to the side of it rather than in alignment.

## INTENSE SIDE STRETCH - PARSVOTTANASANA

PARSVOTTANASANA Is a forward stretch over the front leg with the hands in prayer position behind the back. Firstly, we'll instruct an easier version.

Take a wide stance on the mat stepping your left leg back, the left foot at an angle. Point your right foot forwards. Breathe in, clasp your hands behind your back.

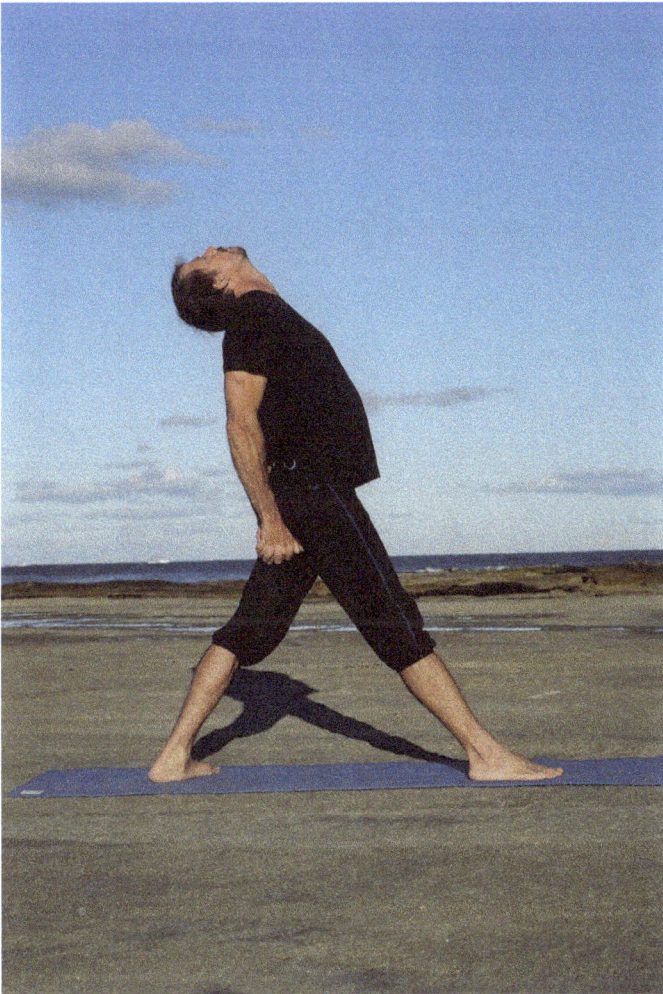

Angle the left hip and the torso forward to face your front leg and foot (in this case the right leg) so that both your hips are angled that way - towards the short end of the mat. Press down with the heels and toes, particularly the base of the big and little toes, to stabilise the feet. Push back the right leg and right side of your body slightly, to help even the hips.

On your next inhalation, extend the trunk upwards and arch back, opening the chest. Breathe out and take the body forward parallel to the mat.

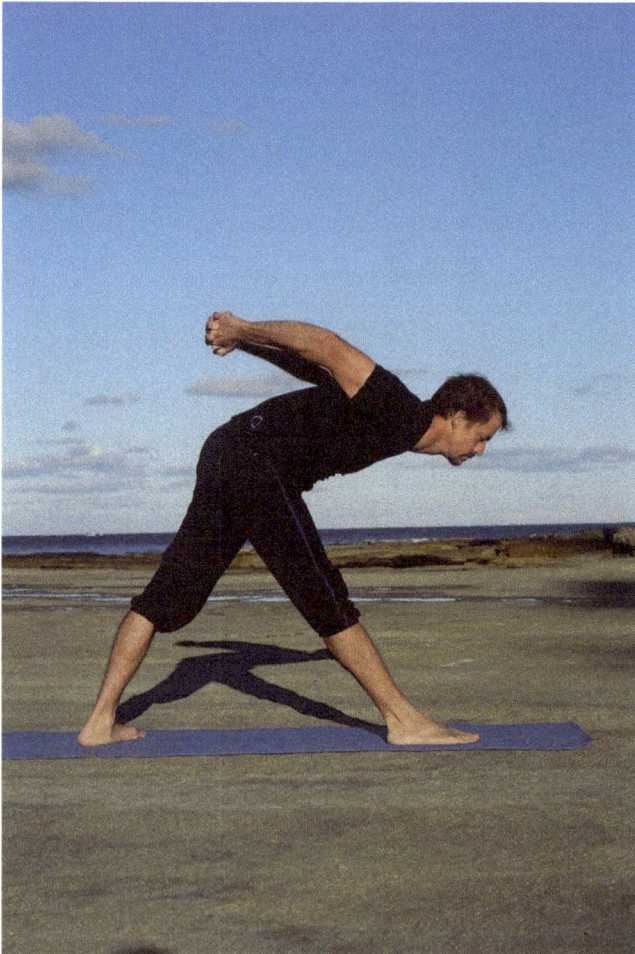

This is adequate for beginner. To extend into a deeper stretch, keeping a long straight back, allow the body to go towards the leg, aiming towards the little toe edge of the leg. Ultimately, if possible, rest the chest on the thigh.

Slowly come up and release the hands.

Change sides so that now your left foot is forward and your right foot is the back foot, slightly at an angle. Restabilise the feet, clasp your hands behind your back, shoulder blades eased towards each other. Breathe in, stretch back and repeat all the steps above. This posture opens the shoulders and stretches the hamstrings, both of which will help increase your mobility.

To do this posture with the hands in reverse prayer behind the back, limber up the arms and wrists first with shoulder exercises.

See the shoulder rolls and the lower shoulder muscles stretches, in Section 1. Also rotate the wrists back and forth.

## INTENSE SIDE STRETCH - PARSVOTTANASANA

Assume we are still working with the right foot forward and left foot being the back foot. Take the wide leg stance as described above, with the hips facing the right/front foot. This time bring the fingertips together behind the back.

Slowly press the whole of the fingers together, then the palms, so that the heels of the hands are together and the fingers pointing upwards in between the shoulder blades. Bring the entire palm and all fingers together evenly, paying attention to the index finger and thumbs.

Ease the hands further upward between the shoulder blades.

Angle the back/left hip forward to face your right foot. Push back the right leg and right side of your body slightly. Extend the body upwards, pulling the lower part of the body in towards the trunk as well as up.

Take the head back and breathe in. Breathe out and stretch forward with a long back. Bring the back parallel to the mat, initially. Extend towards your leg if you're able to maintain length through the back. Continue deep breathing as you hold the posture for approximately six seconds plus.

Inhale and come up, release the hands, then turn both feet to the long edge of the mat. Now turn your left foot to be your front foot and stabilise the right foot to be the back foot. Turn your hips to face your left foot.

Proceed in the same way, this time tucking your left thigh and the left side of the body back and the right hip and thigh forwards to your front/left foot. After holding the pose for the same length of time, breathing freely, inhale and come up, release the prayer stretch or alternative clasp.

Now turn both feet towards the long edge of the mat.

## WARRIOR I - VIRABHADRASANA I

Stand up straight in TADASANA, the mountain pose - with the legs and feet together.

Breathe in and take the arms straight up either side of the ears. Step your legs wide apart with the right foot forward and body facing the right foot.

The left foot will be at a slight angle towards the right one.

On your next exhalation, bend your right knee and take it forward, to a right-angle, with the shin straight and the thigh parallel to the mat. If on stepping forward, the foot is not quite

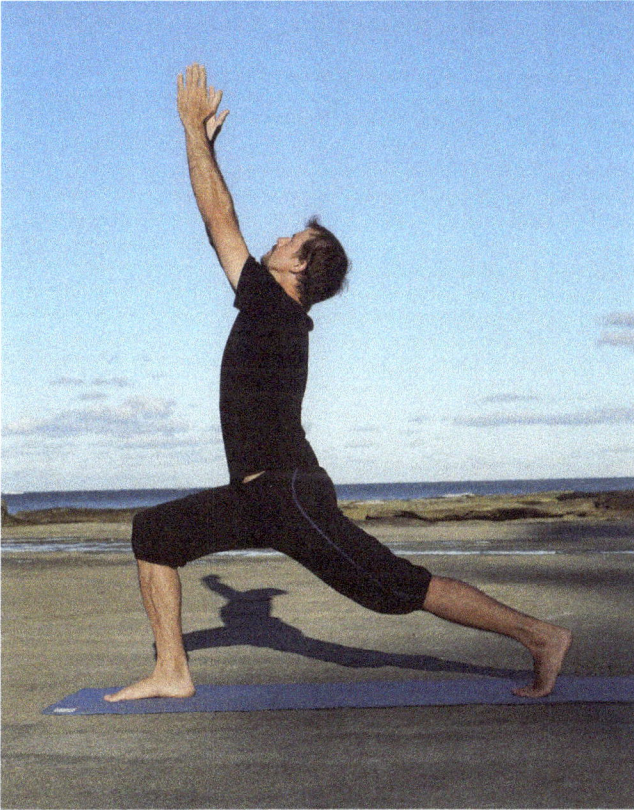

in alignment, as above, ease the foot forward until the leg is vertical. Have the hips facing the same way as your right/ front foot, by easing your right hip slightly back.

If there is no discomfort in the back, extend the stretch and join the hands in prayer position.

Ground down through the feet and keep the hips square to the right toe and short edge of the mat. The back foot will be at an angle.

Another option is to place the legs wide apart to start with, before raising the arms. Still turn the right foot forward, the left foot at a slight angle and square the hips towards the front foot.

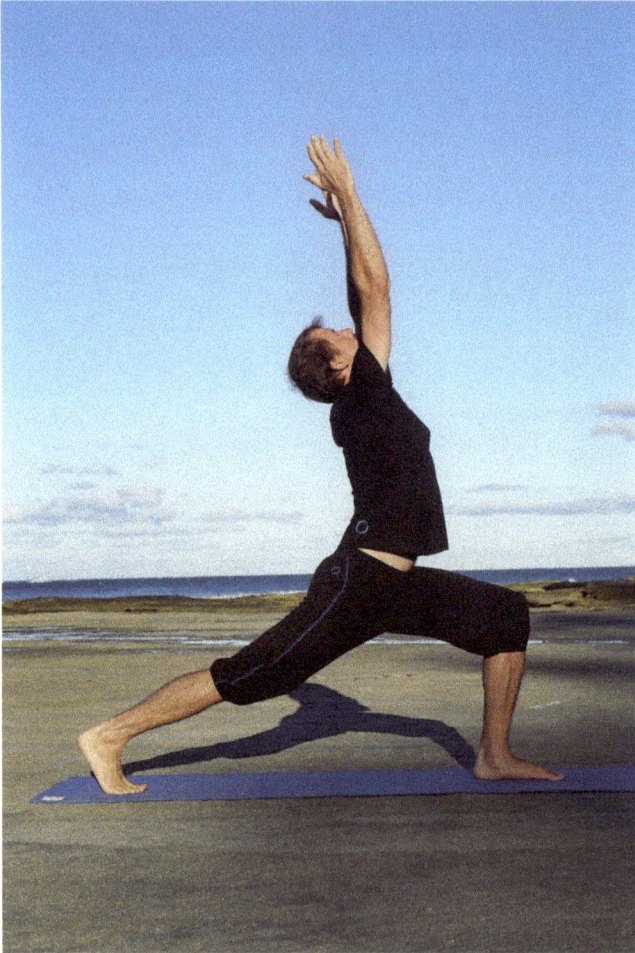

The inner arms should be facing the ears and the palms facing each other, or palms together, but cross the thumbs, or interlace the fingers together and point the index finger up.

Keep the shoulders relaxed and the chest and sternum lifted. Stretch the head back and look towards the hands. Maintain for a few seconds, free breathing.

The posture is good for balance and strengthens the ankles, knees and hips.

To come out of the pose, on the out breath, release the arms down and straighten the front leg.

As this is a strong back stretch, before you change sides, pivot to the left, face the long side of your mat, both feet forward, legs wide apart, and allow the back to soften and fold gently forward from the hips into:

## WIDE-LEGGED STANDING FORWARD BEND - PRASARITA PADOTTANASANA

With the legs wide, fold forward from the hips. Place the hands on the floor either side of your head, shoulder width apart.

Lengthen and stretch the torso forward. A block can be used in order to rest the crown of the head. After taking a few relaxing breaths, straighten the arms and lengthen the back. Breathe in and come up into a standing posture. Alternatively, roll up vertebra by vertebra.

After slowly coming up, turn the left foot forward ready to repeat the posture on this side. After completing this posture on the second side, repeat the forward fold and hold for a few seconds.

## WARRIOR II - VIRABHADRASANA II

Begin in TADASANA. Step the left leg back. Have the legs as wide apart as is comfortable.

Turn the right foot towards the short edge of the mat, but keep the hips facing the long side of the mat. Turn your left foot in, slightly on an angle.

Inhale and bring the arms up to shoulder level parallel to the floor. Reach out through the finger tips, as if stretching towards each wall. Exhale and bend the right knee in a lunge so that the knee is over the ankle. Have the arch of the back foot in line with the heel of the front foot.

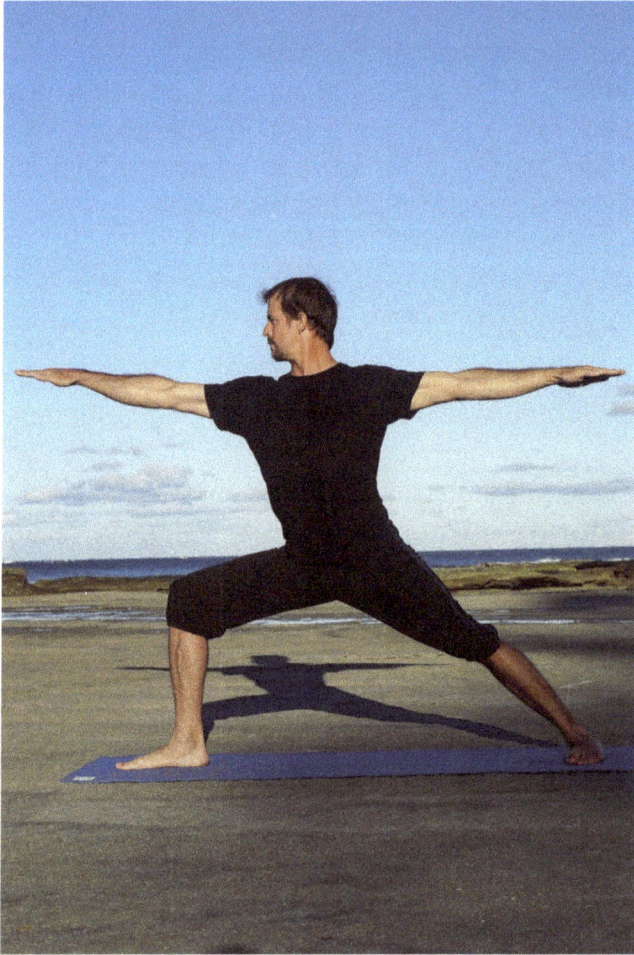

Some traditions advocate heel in line with heel. See which gives you the better alignment. Bend your left hip joint, at the level of the thigh, outward, or tighten the left buttock outwards to the space behind you. This will correct the slight 'lean' forward, shown here.

The body should be vertical. Compare with the following picture.

Turn the head to gaze in the direction of your front foot but look at the right middle finger. Keep the crown of the head up to lengthen through the spine. Press down and 'ground' the feet, keeping the legs strong. Sink the hips down towards the floor, making sure the knee stays over the ankle. Relax the shoulders down and back, the chest out.

Hold the posture for a few deep breaths then bring the arms down by your sides. Straighten the front leg and turn both feet forward to the long edge of the mat. Now prepare to change sides simply turning your left foot out to the short edge of the mat on your left side. Place the right foot as the strong, back foot at a slight angle.

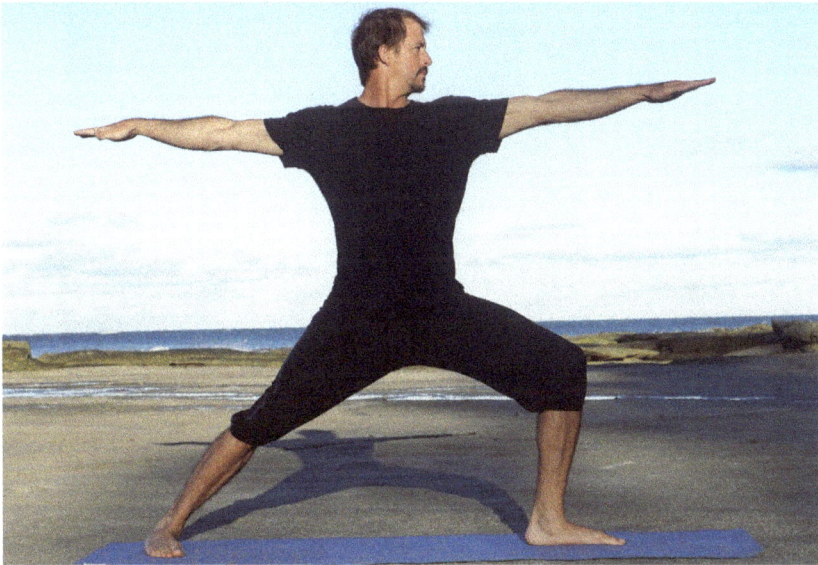

Again, align the arch of the back foot with the heel of the front foot. Repeat the steps on this side. Note the back hip on this side has been adjusted to create a vertical trunk.

When you have completed the second side, walk or jump your feet together. Alternatively, from warrior pose, you can drop the front elbow to the knee and raise the back arm, as depicted.

Warrior II opens the hips and chest and strengthens the legs and body.

## EXTENDED SIDE ANGLE POSE
## - UTTHITA PARSVAKONASANA

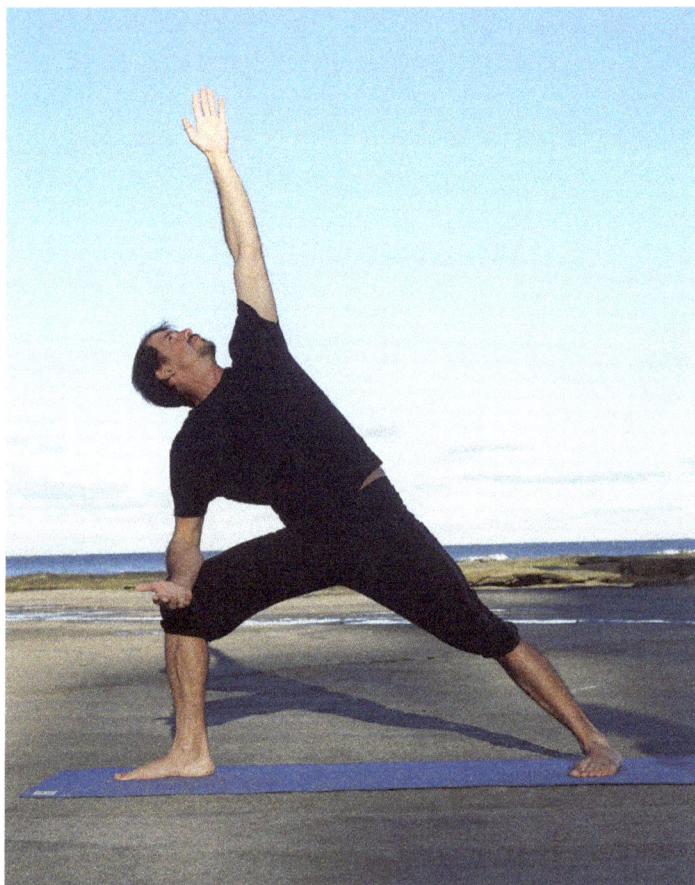

The above is one version of UTTHITA PARSVAKONASANA. You can easily move into this posture from warrior II above.

Simply take the right elbow to your right thigh, (when doing the warrior pose with the right leg forward) as above.

This is a gentler and preparatory option of the full pose, where the body is positioned as described below.

For attempting the full posture, see below:

## EXTENDED SIDE ANGLE POSE
## - UTTHITA PARSVAKONASANA

Begin as for the previous posture, warrior II, then lean your body sideways towards your front thigh.

To begin the pose from the beginning, you would start in TADASANA then step the legs wide apart, facing the long side of your mat with straight legs wide apart. Open your left shoulder, ribs and pelvis. Press weight into the outer edge of your back/left foot.

Turn your right foot out, toes pointing to the short edge of the mat. Exhale bending the right knee so that the thigh is at a right-angle, your knee above the ankle. As above, lean and extend the trunk sideways over the right leg.

Take the right hand to the outer edge of the right foot and place it on the floor outside the little-toe edge of the foot. The back foot should be very slightly angled towards the front foot, as before. Have the arch of the front foot in line with the heel of the back/left foot.

Straighten the right arm. It should be pressed against the right leg. Extend closer to the front leg. Take a few deep breaths. Raise the left arm, palm forward, opening the left side upwards.

When attempting each pose individually and slowly, as opposed to moving through a series of poses together, I would suggest you aim to have the front heel in line with the arch of the back foot for all poses. However, when moving through a series of poses one after the other, heel in line with heel seems to work well. Whichever you choose, be consistent.

Ground the left foot actively into the floor, particularly the little toe edge. Keep the spine and neck long and look straight ahead.

To extend further, sweep your left arm over your head, palm down towards your face, the arm close to your ear. Extend from the outside of the left heel to the left fingertips.

Once in position, turn the head to look up towards the underside of the upper arm and beyond - neck permitting.

To come up: inhale and straighten the right leg. Breathe out and lower the arms, or simply rest them as you come up. Repeat on the other side.

## WARRIOR III - VIRABHADRASANA III

Start off in the mountain pose, then step the legs wide apart as in the previous two poses. Breathe in and bring the arms up close to the head, hands into prayer.

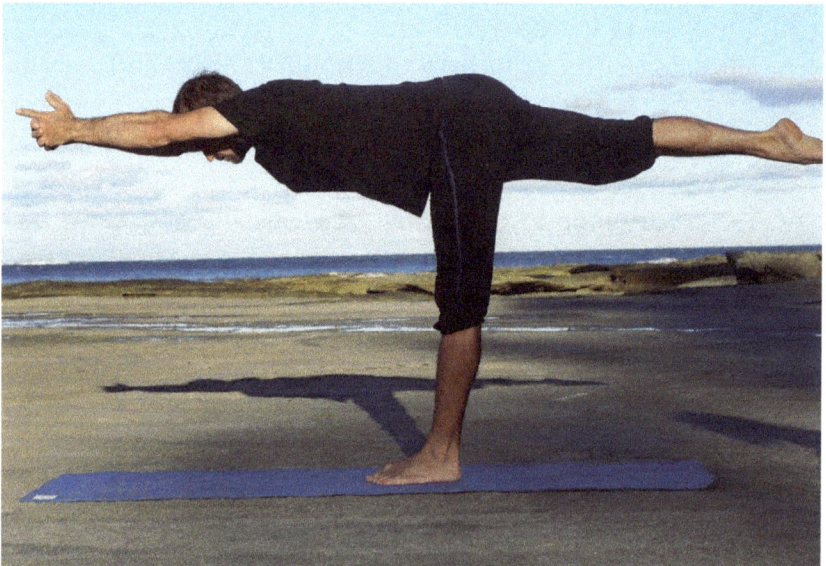

Face the right foot out towards the short edge of the mat and exhale, bending the right knee. Stretch your trunk over your front thigh.

If new to this pose, you may begin without taking the arms out in front of you. In this case, once the knee is over the ankle and you have balance, then bring the arms forward in front of you with the hands in prayer. Alternatively, for beginners or those with challenging balance: try the arms out at the sides at first, like wings, then stretch ahead without the hands being joined.

Ground the right foot into the mat. Exhale, and raise the left leg up, heel towards the sky. In tandem with this movement, straighten the front leg so that the hips and torso are angled towards the floor and are level with the raised leg.

As with other standing poses, focus on a non-moving point. In this case, your face is parallel to the mat, so look down at a fixed point on the floor. Stretch through the left toes and the crown of the head to make a straight line.

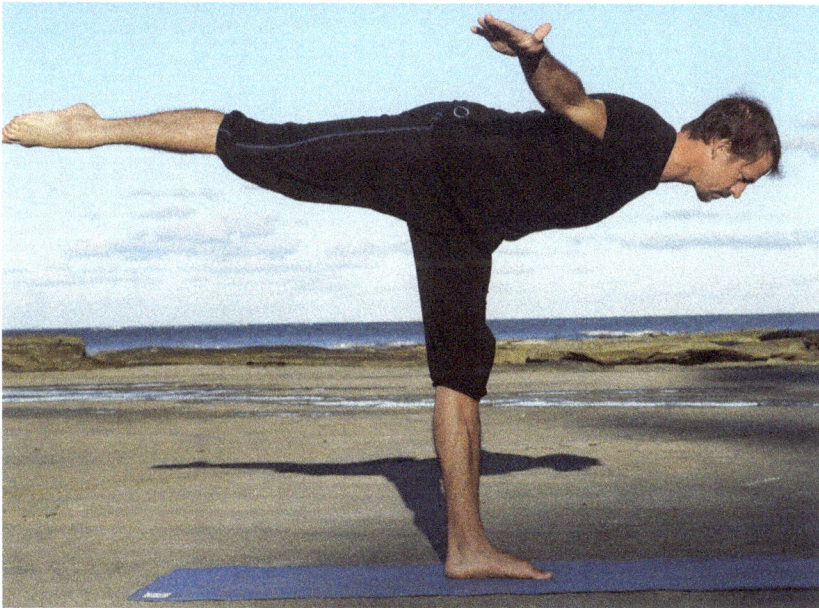

Hold for a few deep breaths. To come out of the pose, inhale taking the arms up, bend the right knee and lower the back leg to the floor. Finally, straighten the legs and step both feet together back into mountain pose.

Repeat on the other side.

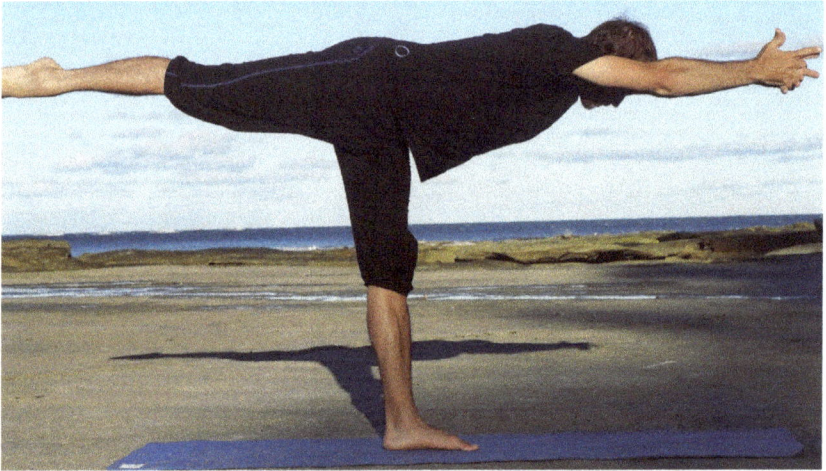

Warrior III improves balance, memory and concentration.

## THE TREE - VRIKSHASANA

Stand up straight with the feet together. You will be bending and raising the right leg and standing on the left. First, ground the left/standing foot into the mat by spreading the toes and broadening through the foot for balance. Imagine the standing foot as a tripod with two points at the front and one at the back.

Raise the right leg. To warm up, rotate the ankle both ways a few times. Next, rotate the knee both ways. To open the hip joint, take your bent leg out as if it were a rural gate. Now you are ready to place that foot on the thigh of the standing leg.

Bend the leg, and place the sole of your right foot against your left thigh.

If possible, bring the sole against the inner thigh of the standing leg and press the heel into the inner groin, toes pointing down. The foot should align with the mid-line of your pelvis.

Bring your hands into the prayer position, first on the breastbone. The shoulders should be down and back and the chest pressing forward.

When you have gained balance, breathe in and raise the arms above the head. Bring the palms together in prayer and interlace the thumbs.

Take several deep breaths in and out through the nose. Hold the posture for 10 seconds, or for as long as you're able. Fix the gaze on something non-moving a few metres in front of you, either on the wall or the floor. Focus your attention.

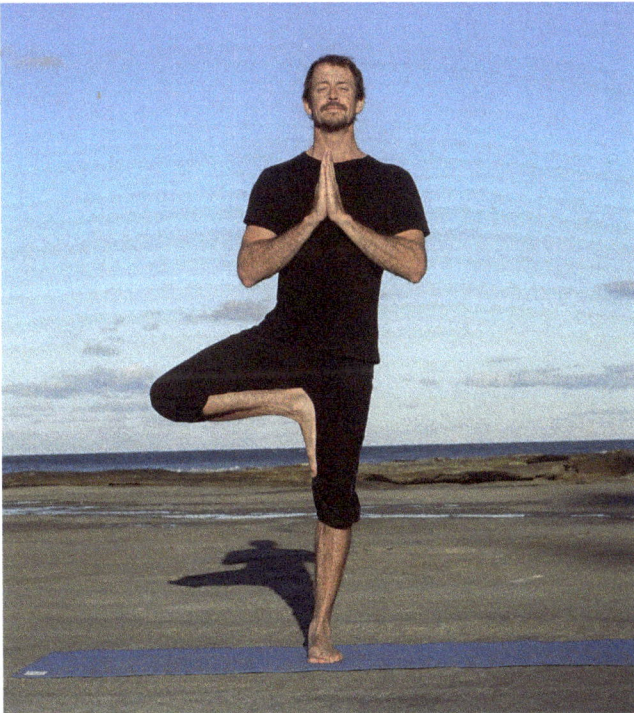

Slowly lower the leg. Repeat on the other side, first rotating the ankle knee and hip, as before, prior to bringing the foot to the thigh.

The posture strengthens the ankles, calves, thighs and spine and it stretches groins. The tree posture also improves your focus, concentration and your balance - within and without.

## THE PENCIL POSE
## (Also known as THE TREE - VRIKSHASANA II)

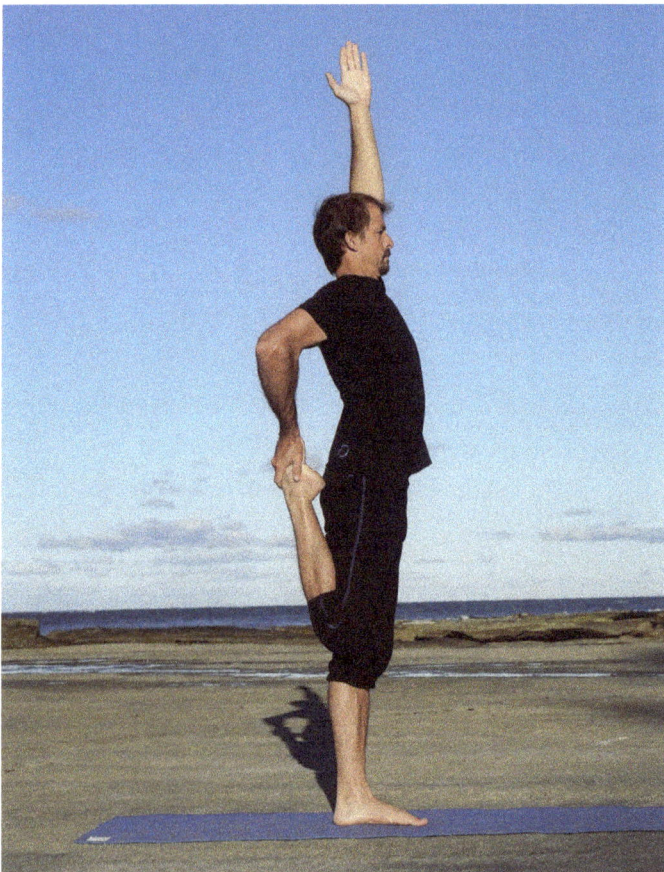

Stand up straight. Place the weight on the standing foot.

Let's assume you are beginning with the left foot. Ground the foot as before. Bend the right calf behind you and draw it close to the body so that the heel goes to the buttock. The thighs are still touching. Breathe in and stretch the opposite arm up, close to the ear, in a line. Have the fingers straight.

Breathe out and release the arm and leg. Change legs and repeat on the other side. Don't lock the standing knee.

This pose is good preparation for the dancer - NATARAJASANA.

## POSE OF THE DANCER - NATARAJASANA

Stand on the left foot.

You can begin with the thighs together as for the last posture. Now bend the right leg from the knee, take it behind you and hold the foot.

Breathe in, taking this leg upwards and back. Have your right thumb on the outside of the foot.

Raise your left arm out in front of you. Gain your balance then take your right foot up so that the calf is stretched upwards and the thigh is away from the body. Draw it backwards.

At the same time, hinge forward from the hips. Keep the chest open. Extend the left arm forward, the palm facing forward.

Focus your attention on something non-moving. Maintain for 6-20 seconds, breathing normally.

Exhale and return to a standing position.

Repeat, standing on your right foot, capturing your left foot with the left hand and extending the right hand and arm.

## POSE OF THE DANCER - NATARAJASANA

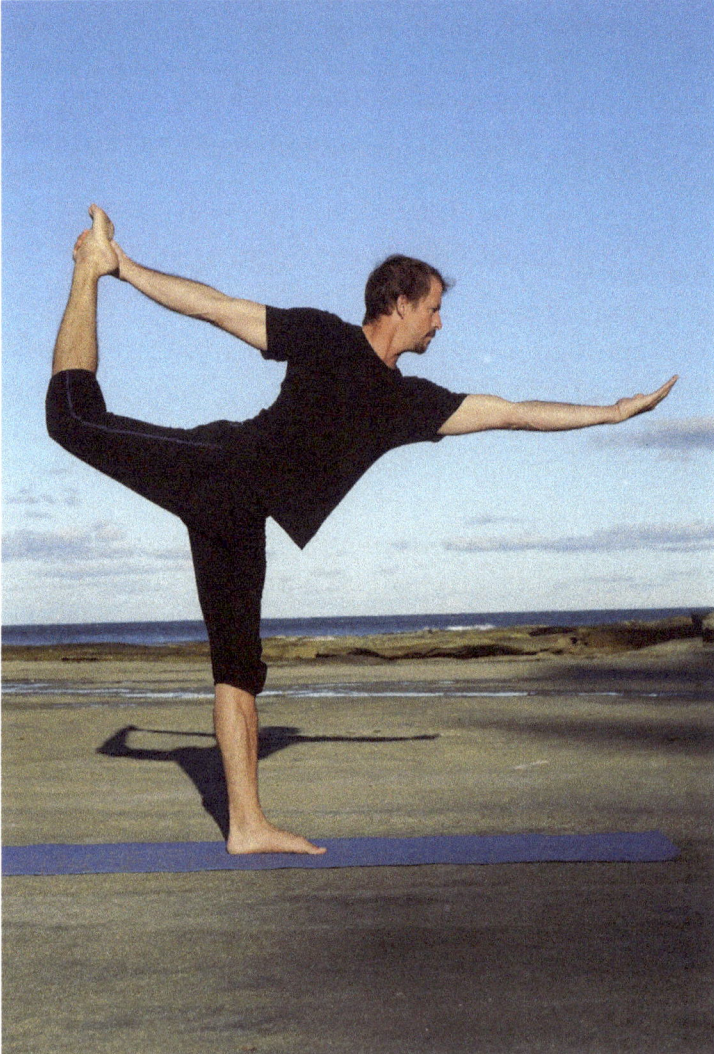

# SECTION 4

## STRONGER STRETCHES AND BACK BENDS

### HALF LOCUST - ARDHA-SALABHASANA

Lie face down with the chin on the ground, legs together, straight, hands by your side.

Make fists with your hands and take them under the tops of the thighs, where the thighs join the hips.

Raise one leg straight up keeping the other one the ground. Hold for a few seconds, then on an exhalation, lower the leg. After a few seconds rest, raise the other leg, hold and release. After the pose, turn your head to one side and rest for a few breaths.

### THE LOCUST - SALABHASANA

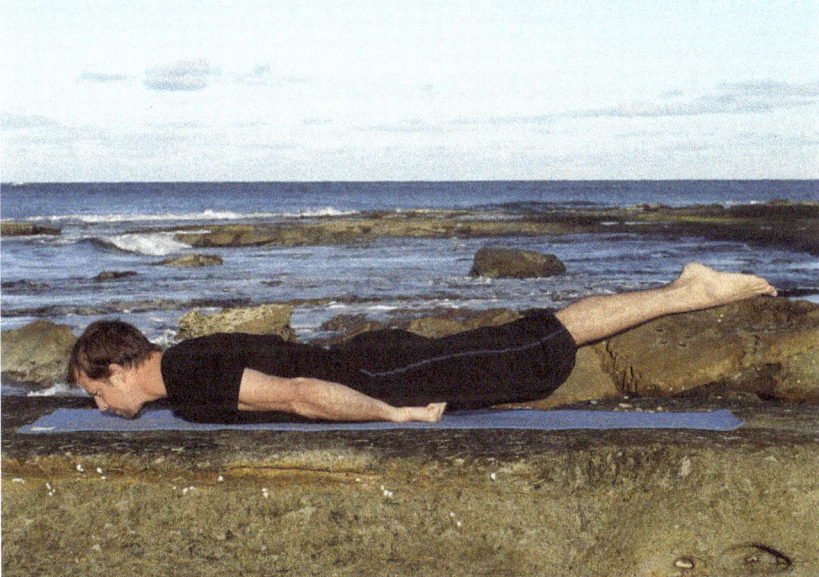

Lie face down with the chin on the ground, legs together, straight, hands by your side. Firstly, make fists with your hands and take them under the tops of the thighs, where the thighs join the hips.

Breathe in, and on an out breath, raise the legs, open your palms and help push up the legs. The photo on the previous page depicts this warm-up method. Beginners may keep their foreheads on the mat, rather than the chin. Modify to suit.

The full asana requires the fists in the groin but the backs of the hands kept on the mat and the legs raised without assistance.

The hands can also be palm down by the sides of your hips, with the thumbs facing the edges of the mat. If trying this option, press the palms down into the mat.

After the posture, gently lower the legs and turn your head to one side.

## THE BOAT - NAVASANA

There are many versions of NAVASANA. The following is easily achieved.

Lie on the stomach with the legs stretched out as straight as possible. More flexible or experienced students should bring the legs close together.

Clasp your hands behind your hips.

Inhale and raise your upper chest and legs. Your face should be looking forward.

Exhale and lift more through the chest and legs.

Inhale pushing your shoulder blades towards each other. At the same time, stretch your arms and hands back towards your feet.

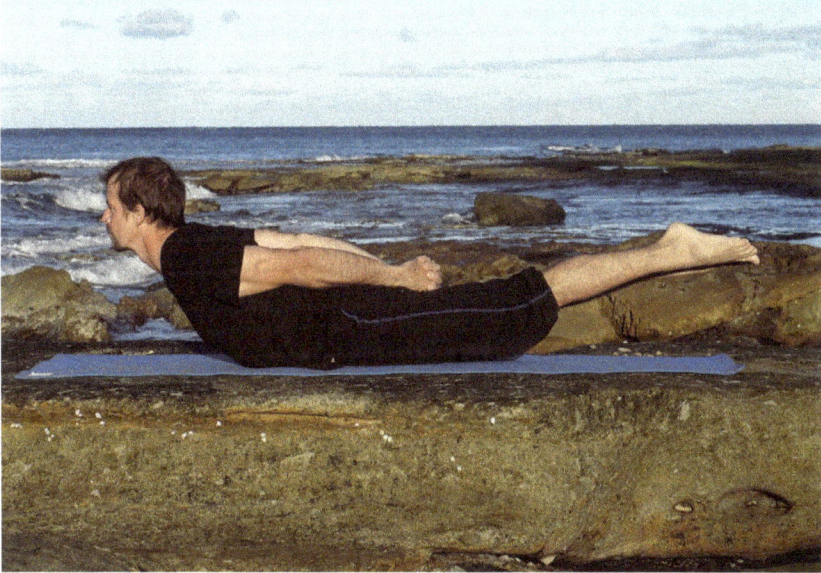

Weight should rest on the middle of your body so that you are balancing on the stomach muscles. Reach back through the balls of your feet.

Take several deep breaths in and out as you hold the pose for several seconds.

Then, on an exhalation, lower your body back to the mat. Turn your head the opposite way from the last resting pose - with the other side of your head on the mat.

The above posture strengthens the back muscles and ligaments, restores mobility to sacroiliac region and helps prevent backache. It stimulates the adrenal glands, cleanses and rejuvenates the kidneys, expands the chest and helps firm the arms and bust or chest.

NAVASANA can also be practised with the arms on the mat. Thumbs towards the two outside edges of your mat and the little fingers nearest to the body.

## THE BOW - DHANURASANA

Lie on the stomach, face down and legs on the mat.

Breathe in and as you breathe out bend the knees so that the calves are bent towards you. The legs can be close together or about hip distance apart at the knees. Grasp your ankles with your hands and have the thumbs, fingers and back of the hand on the outside of the ankles. Bring your feet as close as you can to your buttocks.

With the chin on the floor, breathe in, raise the head and shoulders and ease your thighs off the mat, stretching your heels towards the ceiling. Press your shoulder blades firmly in and draw the shoulders back. The elbows should be straight.

Grasping the ankles strongly, lift the legs up, and 'bow' back, balancing on the stomach. If you have difficulty, widen the legs slightly more. You will discover, holding this pose and breathing deeply and rhythmically in and out through the nose, that as you breathe in and out the body may gently rock on the stomach/hips with the breath.

Stabilise your body to hold the pose for a few seconds. Breathe out and slowly lower yourself to the floor. With strong back-bends such as this, it is advisable to then come onto your knees and sit back on the heels in the pose of the child.

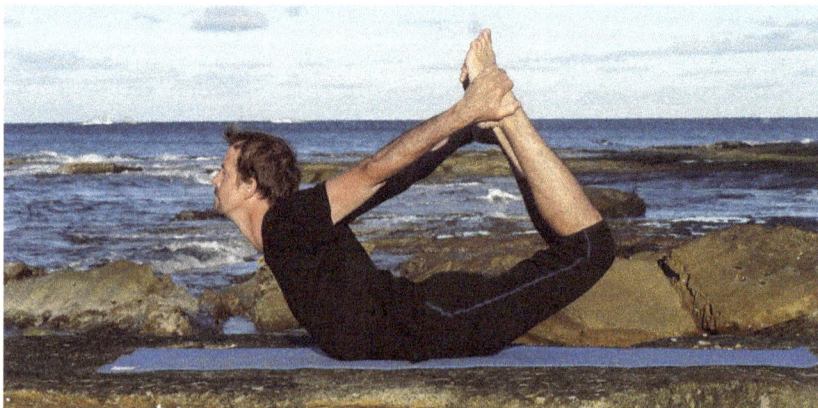

The bow posture strengthens the spinal muscles and tones the kidneys and adrenals.

If this is not an achievable posture for you, try firstly holding your ankles, breathing in and just raising the upper body. Keep the thighs on the ground. Breathe out and lower.

Now place the forehead on the mat. Breathe in, then as you breathe OUT, raise only the thighs. This will be much harder. They may only lift slightly. Keep the upper body down.

Relax, and then re-try the full posture, grasping your ankles and raising the face, upper body and legs on the inhalation. Exhale, release, and come into pose of the child BALASANA.

## THE CAMEL - USTRASANA

*NOTE: Not to be attempted where there are vertebral disc issues.*

Kneel upright on your mat.

Traditional yoga has the knees and ankles placed together. For experienced or flexible students this can be attempted. Otherwise, it will be best to begin with the knees hip width apart.

To get the feel of the posture, place the hands on the hips with the thumbs angling towards the spine. Press the thumbs into the muscles either side of the spine below the waist, about half-way up the lower back/ the back of the hips. Arch back, pushing the shoulder blades together.

Massage the lower back forward with the thumbs, pushing the hips out. Gradually walk the thumbs a little higher towards the waist and arch back more.

Return to the upright kneeling position then drop forward into the pose of the child, BALASANA, for a few seconds, to rest your back.

Slowly come up again ready to attempt the full camel, or simply repeat as above.

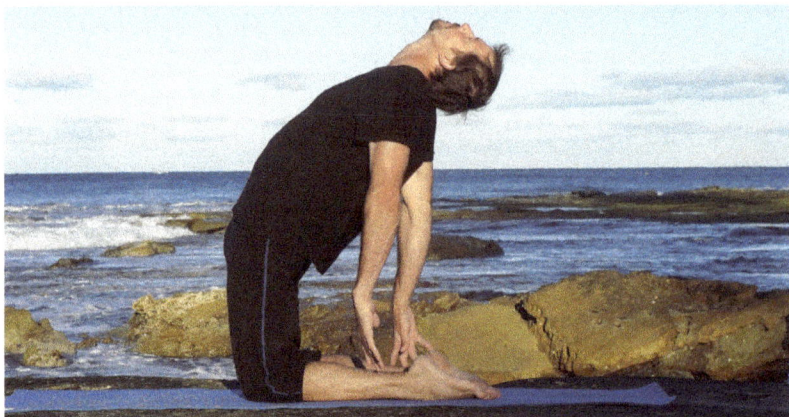

To extend into the full camel, if comfortable, you can reach back with both arms and grasp the ankles with the thumbs on the inside of the ankles. Have the palms hold each heel and your fingers pointing toward your toes.

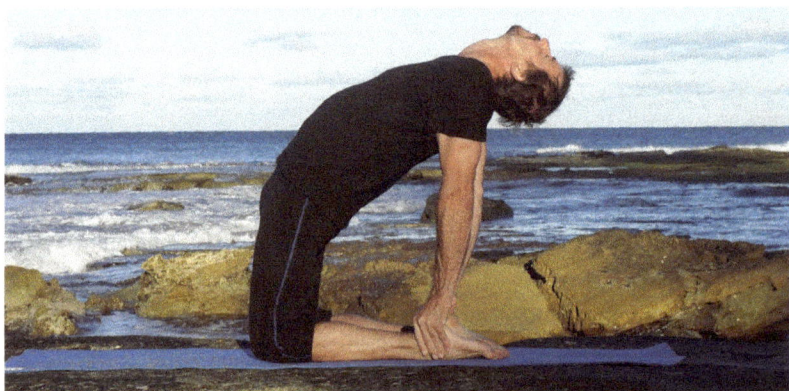

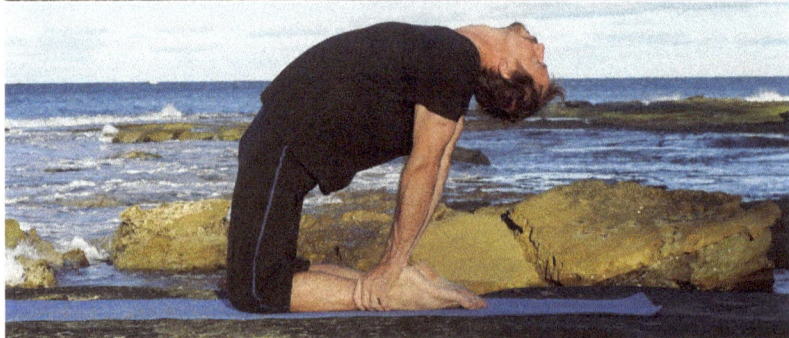

For ease, it often helps to breathe in and take one arm up, and then down in a huge semi-circle, to grasp the heel as you breathe out. Then the other arm.

As soon as you take hold of the ankles, thrust the pelvis forward and drop your head and neck back. Breathe freely in and out through the nose.

Hold for as many seconds as is comfortable.

To release, bring your hands back to your front hips or thighs and resume the upright kneeling posture.

Inhale and take your head and body forward into child's pose, BALASANA, as you exhale.

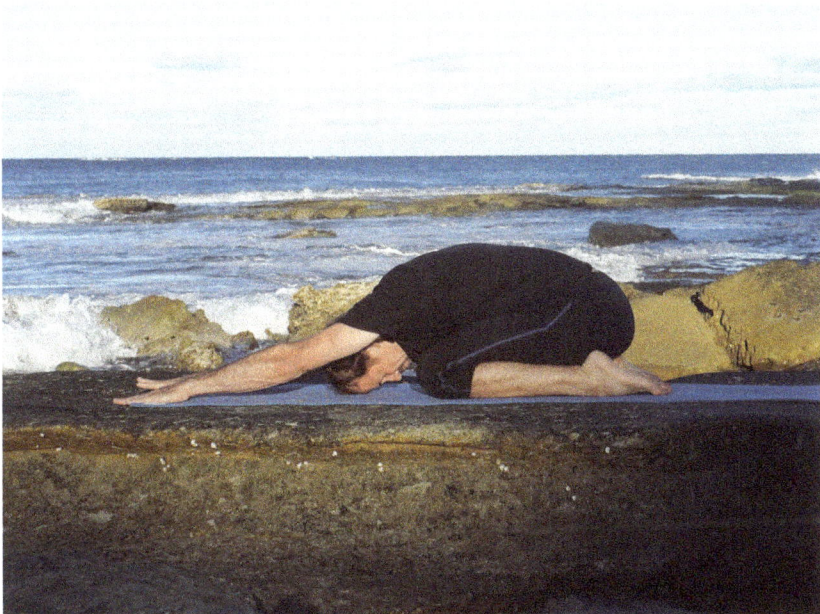

The camel posture strengthens the vertebral column, stretches the front of the body and can correct bad posture.

The kidneys and adrenal glands receive a good massage.

## THE BRIDGE - SETUBANDHASANA/ SETUBANDHA SARVANGASANA

Here, we repeat the bridge posture from Section 1, now followed by an extended stretch over a block.

When using a block, have the block handy by the side of your body, and have your back on the mat.

Bend the knees and place the feet flat to lift the hips up, supporting yourself with your feet on the mat, as in the first bridge posture. Bring your feet under your knees. Once the hips are lifted, take the block tall-way up, if the flexibility of your spine permits, and, place the block under the sacrum -

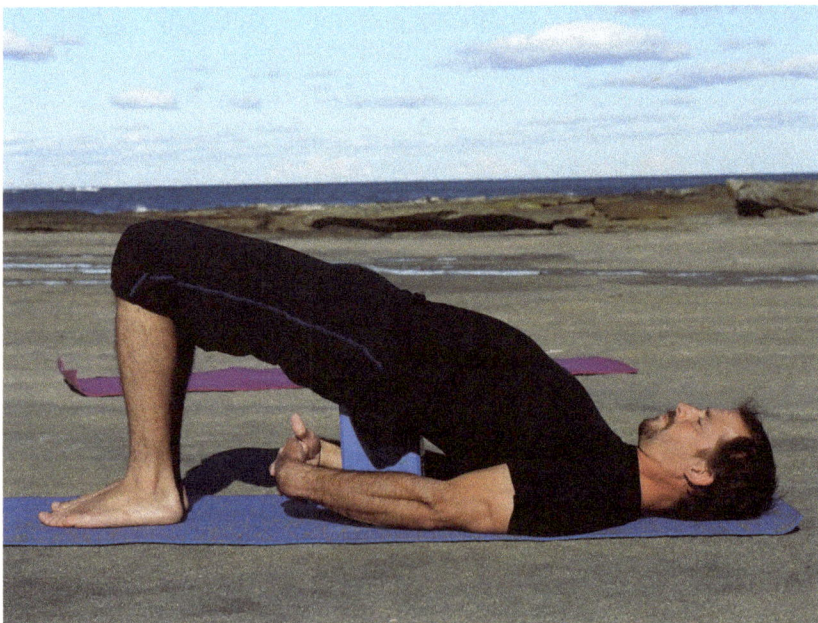

the last few vertebrae of the spine.

Even if you find yourself coming up onto the toes slightly to facilitate placement of the block, the feet should then be placed flat on the floor.

The feet should be firm for stability. Keep the thighs active.

If stable, you can walk your legs out into a straight line, as below, keeping the feet about hip-width distance apart as you extend the legs out in front of you.

Roll the shoulders down into the floor and clasp your hands beyond the block - the foot side of the block; stretch your arms toward your feet. Widen across the collarbones. This is a great stretch for your back and aids good body posture.

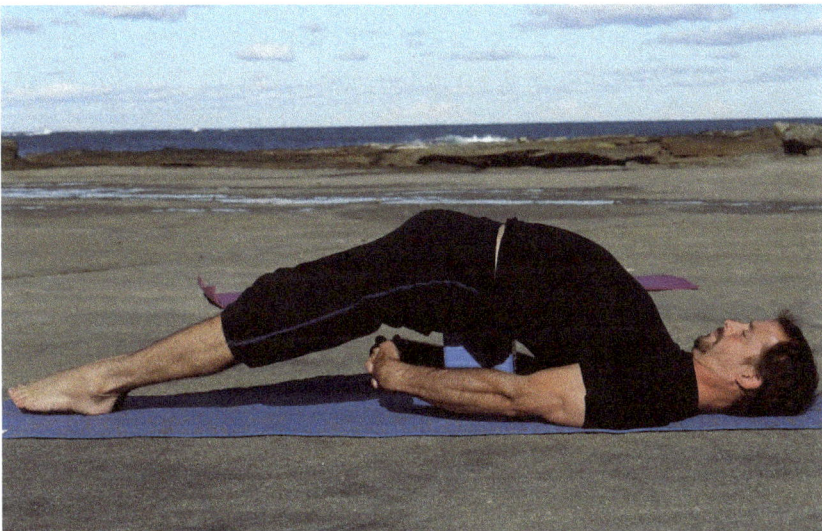

Remove the block and gently lower the back to the mat. After the bridge pose using a block, particularly, make sure you bring the knees up to the chest and roll around hugging your knees to massage the back and spine.

Think of a clock hand. Rock down the left side of your back, across the coccyx, up the right side and across the shoulder blades, several times, then reverse the order, rolling anti-clockwise.

Now rock yourself up into a sitting position.

Students for whom using a block under elevated hips is not appropriate, stick to the bridge posture depicted earlier in Section 1.

For convenience, instructions are summarised here:

Lie on your back with your knees up, feet up to your buttocks on the floor and the feet, knees and ankles hip distance apart.

Press down with the inside of your arms and hands, the balls and heels of your feet, and slowly lift your lower back, hips, middle and upper back off the floor, so that you are resting on your shoulders and feet. There should be no pressure on your neck. Gently ease the shoulder blades inwards. Touch the chest to the chin without bringing the chin down. Both the thighs should be parallel to each other and to the floor. The buttocks and thighs are to be active.

Take a few slow, deep breaths in and out holding the posture. Alternatively, place your hands on your hips and help push up your hips. Have your knees over your ankles and the knees no wider than your hip width. Don't let the legs relax and fall outwards.

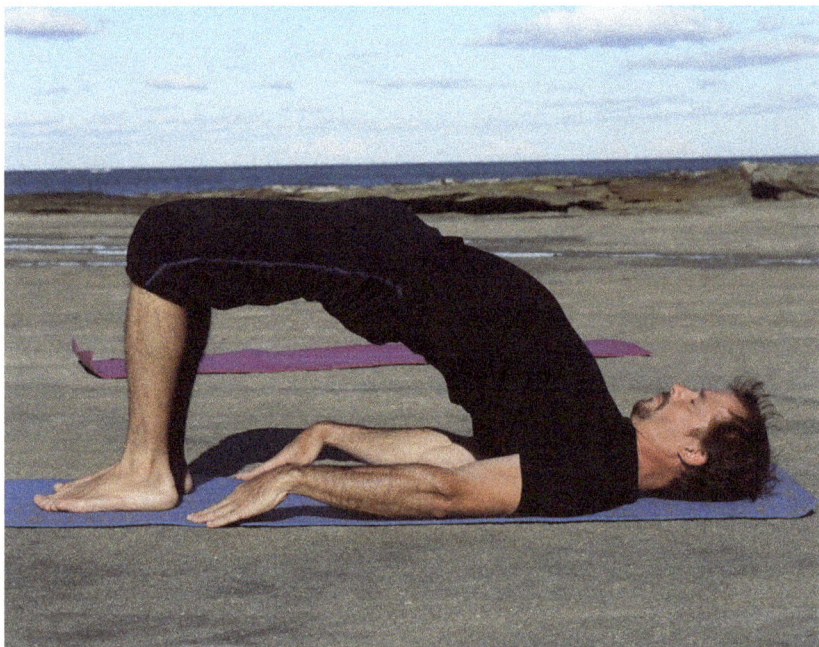

You can also interlace the fingers and push the hands on the floor to lift the torso a little higher. After a few deep breaths, gently lower the shoulder blades, followed by the rest of the body. Bring the knees to the chest and roll around for a few seconds.

## HALF WHEEL POSE - ARDHA CHAKRASANA

Lie on your back, your legs bent.

Bend your elbows and take your hands to the mat at the sides of your head with the fingers pointing towards your shoulders and feet. Rise on your feet and hands, lifting your pelvis.

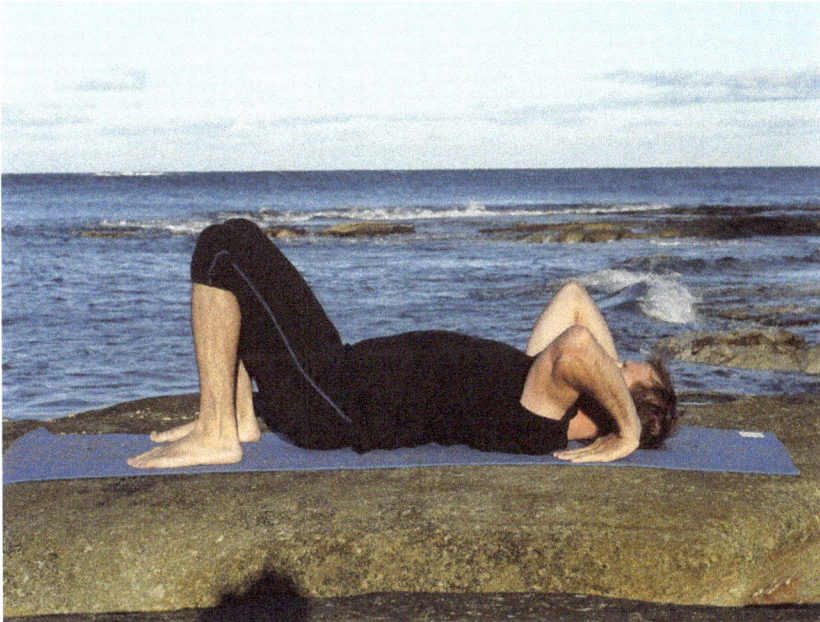

Put the crown of your head on the mat then come down. Repeat a few times holding for a few seconds each time.

## THE WHEEL - CHAKRASANA

Begin in the same way as for the preceding asana - on your back with your legs bent, feet below the buttocks and knees in line with your hips.

Press your palms against the floor at the sides of your head, fingers pointing toward your shoulders and feet. Bend your elbows pointing them upwards. They should only be shoulder width apart. Inhale and anchor the feet firmly into the floor.

As you exhale push the pelvis, hips and trunk up, taking the crown of the head to the floor. Keep your feet approximately hip width apart, thighs and feet parallel.

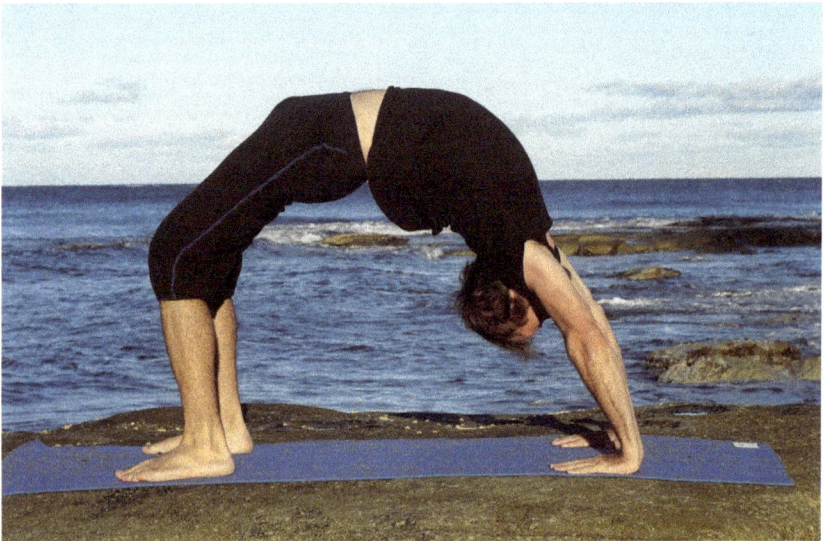

Inhale and press down firmly with the hands and feet, then exhale and lift the crown off the mat, keeping the arms and elbows parallel. Breathe in then on the exhalation straighten the arms and legs as much as possible so that the hips and chest are pushed up lifting the body higher. The spine should resemble the upper half of a circle or semi-circular wheel supported by the hands and the feet.

Lower gently down onto your back for a few seconds, knees still bent. Take a few breaths then hug your knees to your chest. Roll around like a ball - down one side of your body, across the base of the spine, up the other side, and across the shoulder blades.

The pose strengthens the legs, back, thighs and arms. It massages the whole back and the nerve centres. As with many backbends, the adrenal glands are stimulated. The pituitary and pineal glands in the head receive more blood supply, good for the memory function.

## THE POSTERIOR OR FORWARD STRETCH
## - PASCHIMOTTANASANA

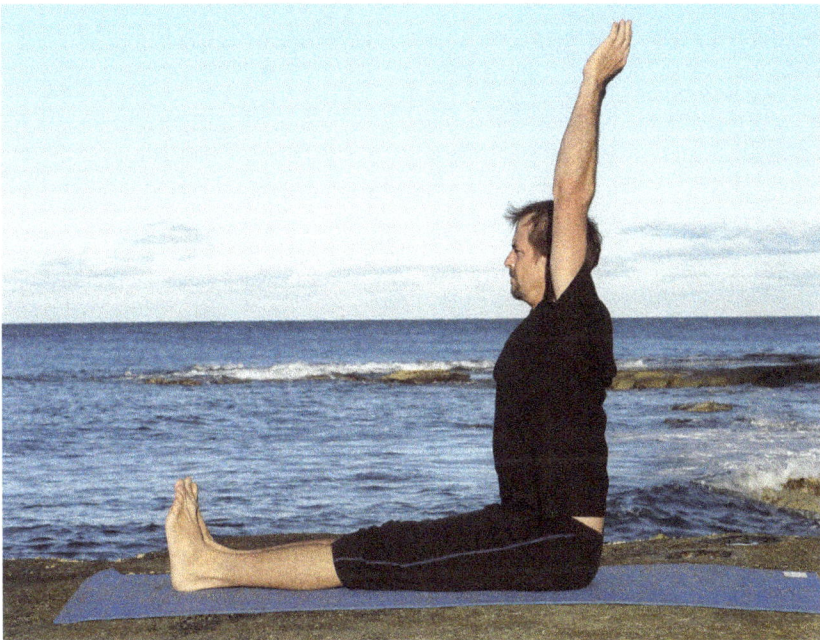

Sit with your legs together stretched out in front of you, the knees soft, not locked. Press down with the hands either side of the body, lift the buttocks then reseat yourself on the front part of the sitting bones.

It helps to walk the buttocks back, one-two, three-four, then lift and re-seat.

Inhale deeply then exhale and extend forward from the hip joints, sliding the hands down the legs towards the feet. Grasp the arches or the ankles.

Draw the inner groin area into the pelvis as you slowly take the lower part of the belly to touch the thighs, then the middle body, ribs and finally the head. Ideally, you will lower your face to your shins. Don't strain to take the head to the shins.

As with all postures, care should be taken if there are any disc injuries or other acute challenges in the body.

Avoid bending the shoulders or hunching just to touch your toes. So, with each inhalation, lift and lengthen the front torso just slightly. With each exhalation, release a little more fully into the forward bend.

As you hold the feet, bend the elbows out to the sides and lift them away from the floor. Lengthen the tailbone away from the back of your pelvis as you ease the front torso lower.

Breathe evenly in the posture for 6 to 30 seconds.

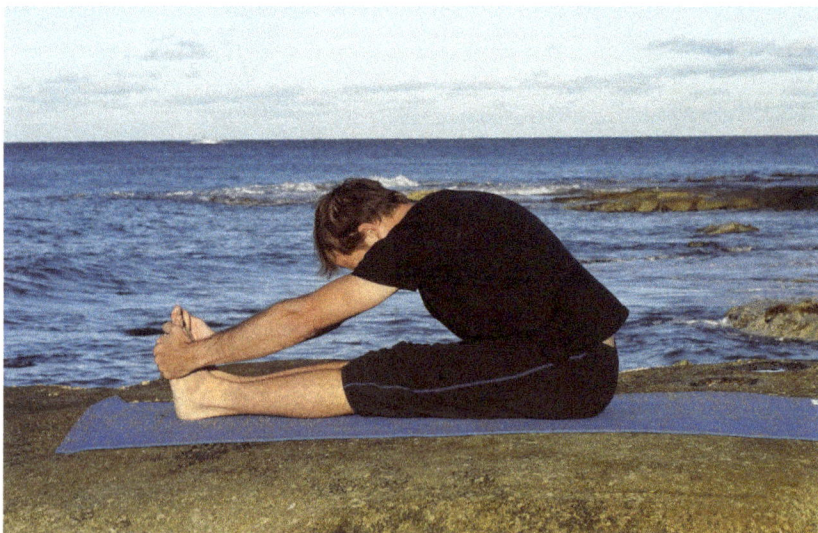

While the aim is the full pose as described, finally grasping your big toes, or wrapping your hands around the feet, it is better to keep a long back and rest the forehead on a cushion on your legs, until you can lower to the thighs in the way described.

As a forward stretch this posture can ease lower back pain and stretch the hamstrings. The full posture has the added benefits of stretching the buttocks and squeezing and toning the abdominal organs. The digestion and function of the intestines can be improved.

The flow of blood to the pelvic region nourishes the bladder and kidneys and tones the reproductive organs.

The intricate web of nerves along the spine are toned. Additionally, the muscles, tendons and ligaments associated with the spine are strengthened, so this posture helps maintain a healthy spine.

## PIGEON POSE - KAPOTASANA

There are other versions of the pigeon pose. This is one of the less strenuous versions, although it can still be challenging.

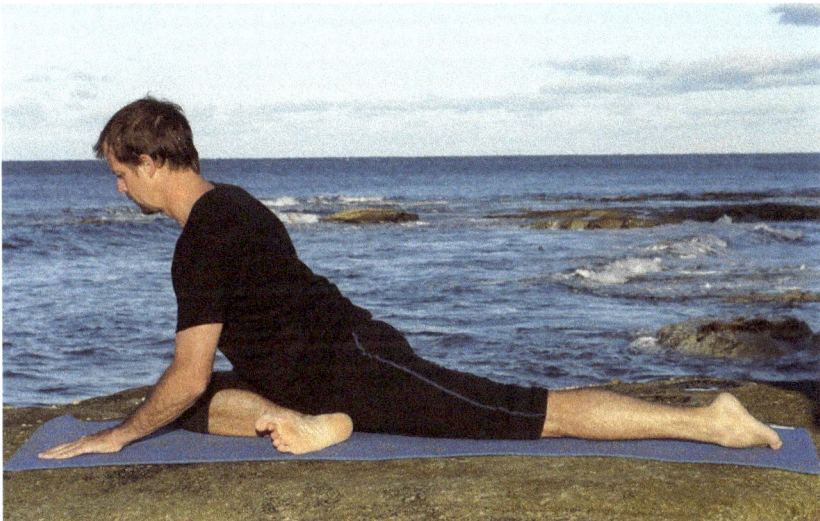

From dog pose, bend your right knee and take the leg forward and place the knee on the mat behind your right wrist with the foot towards your left wrist - across the mat. Another way to begin this pose is on all fours with your hands below your shoulders, knees below your hips. Whichever way you begin, bring your right knee to touch your right wrist.

From this position, keep your hips even and your right thigh parallel to the side of your mat. Bring your right foot just in front of your left hip. If your hips allow, walk your right foot closer to the front of your mat to create a more intense stretch. Many students will find it more comfortable to have the heel close to the hip.

Either way, slide your left leg toward the back of your mat and sink both hips toward the floor. If your right foot is close to the left groin you can roll the groin over the heel of your foot as you settle the hips down. For the full posture, the hips should be even, not rolling to the bent leg side.

For beginners, however, try rolling onto the bent leg side first, for a few breaths, then bring your hips to rest more evenly with the left hip over the right foot.

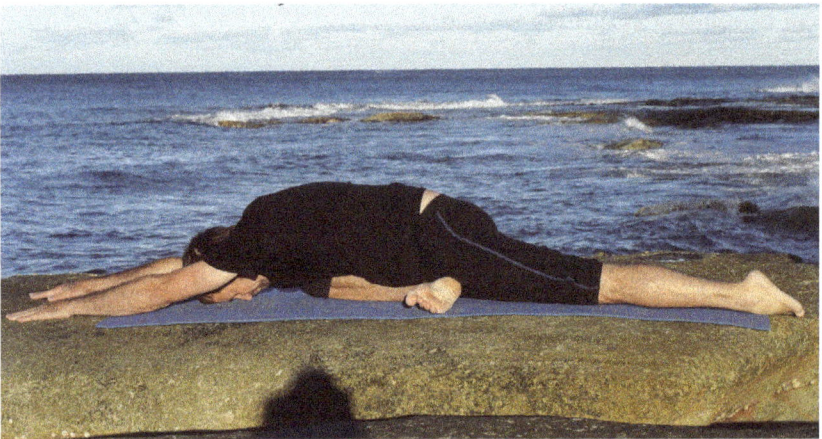

Exhale and bend forward from the hips, sliding the arms and chest onto the mat.

Check your left leg is extended straight out behind you and press the top of your left foot into the mat.

Take a few deep breaths.

To deepen the posture, walk your arms forward until your forehead rests on the floor, stretching and resting the body down.

You can stretch your outer hip more deeply by keeping your elbows off the ground. To stretch the right buttock more, open the right knee more and roll the left hip down towards the floor.

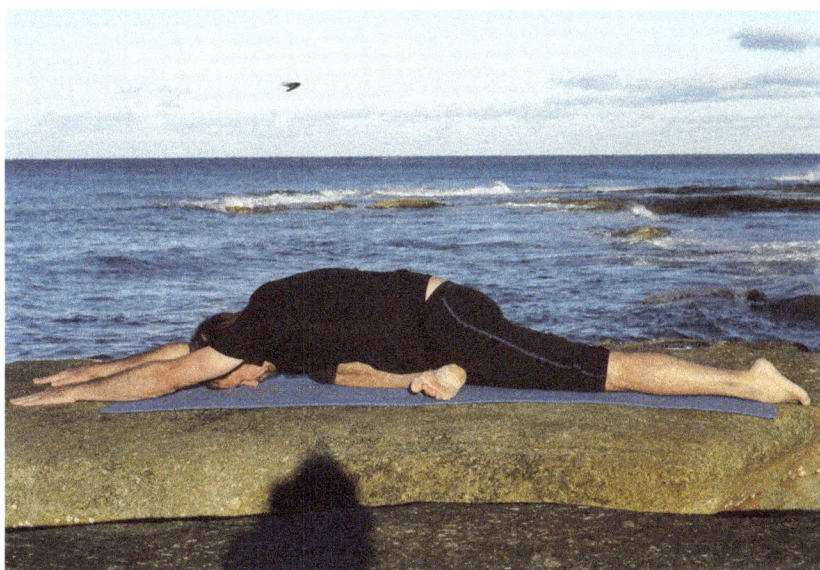

You will feel sensations in the hips and legs. Relax the face as you continue more deep breaths in and out. Release, and before repeating on the other side, try another pigeon variation as below.

If desiring to come out of the posture, press down with the hands and lift the hips to come into cat of dog posture.

## THE LIFTED PIGEON POSE - KAPOTASANA (VARIATION)

From the previous pigeon posture, with the right leg forward, inhale and push down with your hands to raise the upper body. Lift the chest and head.

Have your arms straight by your sides and your hands by your hips, for a few seconds, deep breathing.

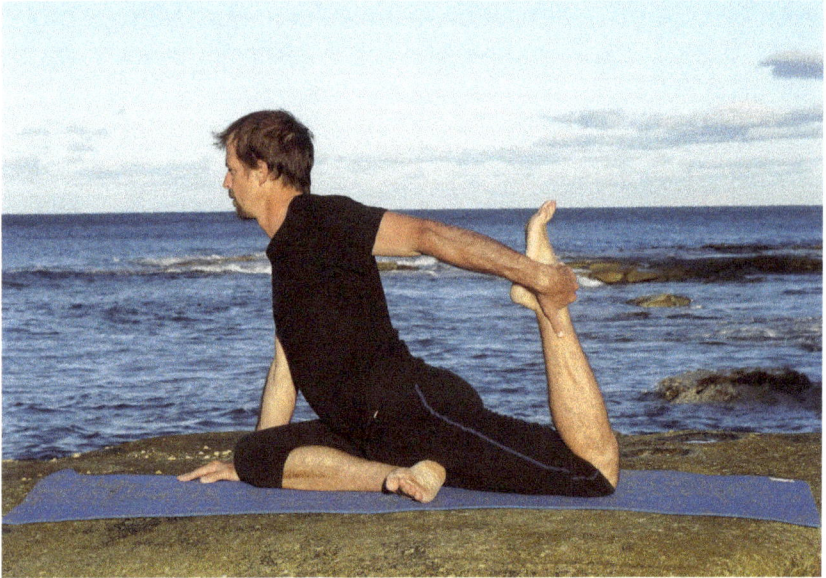

Draw the shoulder blades down, bending slightly back. Keep the left thigh down. Bend your outstretched left leg at the knee and reach back with your left hand and catch your left ankle.

Your right hand will stay on the mat for the moment and your bent right leg will stay the same. The hips should be level. Initially your body may incline more to the right side - the bent leg side; aim to keep the hips even.

Take hold of the outside of your left ankle with the left hand and draw the calf up towards the left buttock. Have the front of the left thigh angled towards the mat. Ease your left foot into the crease of your left elbow.

Maintain equal weight in both hips. Use your core muscles to hold the body steady, then on an inhalation, stretch your right arm up. Exhale and extend it over your head, stretching towards your left hand. Interlace the fingers.

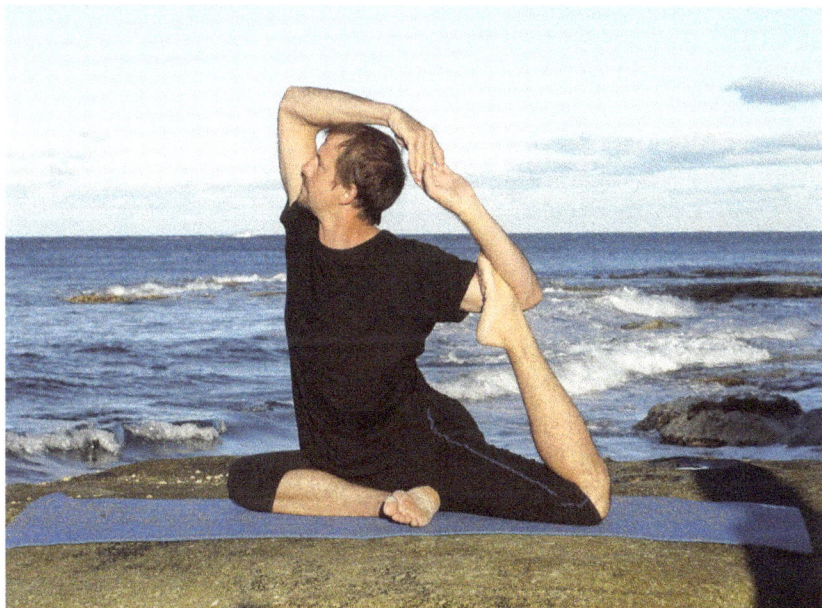

Lift through the ribs to the crown of the head. Hold this variation for four or five deep breaths.

Slowly release and place your hands on either side of your right leg. Let the left leg release and slide back to the mat. Adjust the hands to be either side of your body, tuck the left toes in and bring back the right leg, also tucking the toes into the mat, and lifting the hips into dog stretch. Alternatively, come onto all fours.

Repeat both the first version of the posture, followed by this variation, on the opposite side. To exit from the pigeon posture - KAPOTASANA, release the back leg, press down with your hands either side of the hips and come into the dog stretch, or, onto all fours.

Finally, come into pose of the child.

# SECTION 5

## STRETCHING TOGETHER/PARTNER WORK

---

## FORWARD BEND TOGETHER

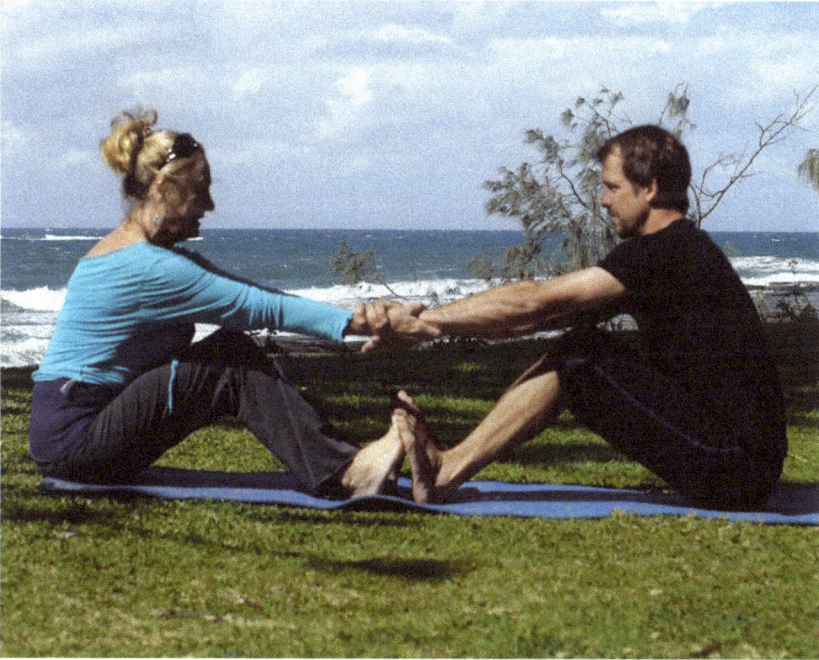

Bring two mats edge to edge and sit facing each other with the feet pressed against the other person's - evenly if possible. Knees may be bent to begin with. Each walk the buttocks back until the legs are as straight as possible.

With different heights, arm and leg length, often one person might have their knees slightly more bent than the other.

Keep the crown of the head up.

Grab each other's wrists, not hands, as this is safer. Breathe in. Use the pull from the other person to lift through the chest taking the crown of the head towards the sky or ceiling so that your sternum lifts and the back lengthens from the tailbone to the crown of the head.

Breathe out, extending into the stretch and stretching the inside of your legs towards your partner's feet.

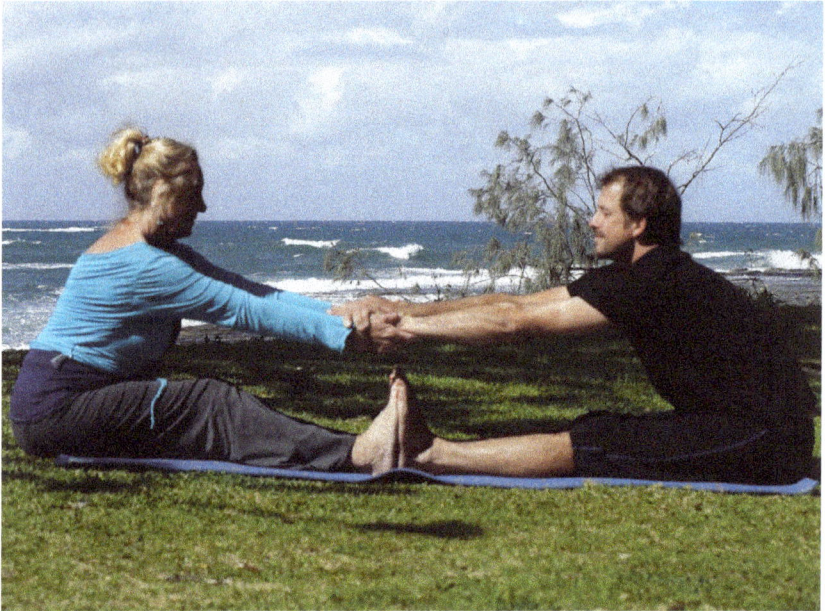

The sciatic nerves are stretched, menstrual and muscular cramps prevented.

## ASCENDING BALANCE

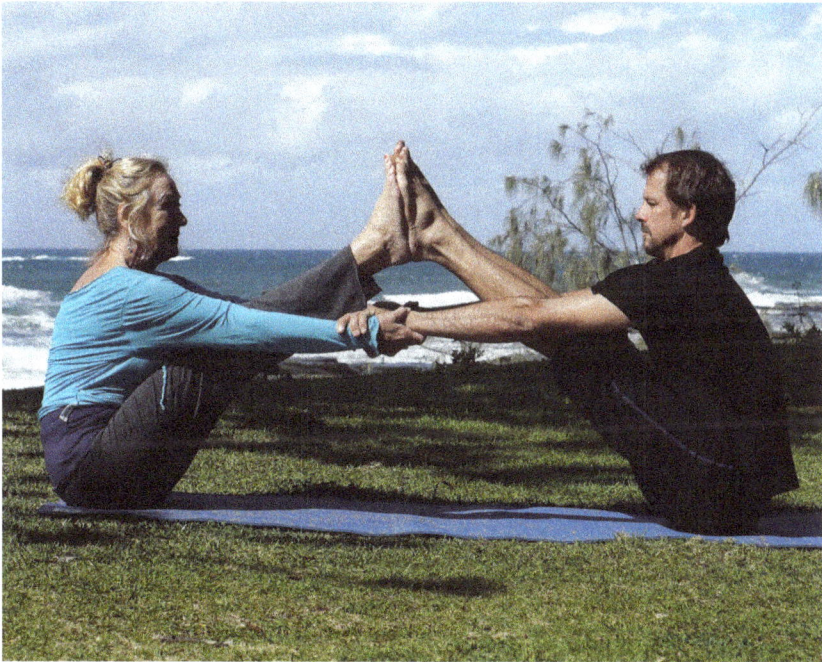

From the previous posture, come a little nearer to each other so that you each have your knees bent and legs close together. You will be pushing against each other's feet and raising the legs. Do this one side at a time. First, decide whose left foot in tandem with the other's right foot, will be the first up. Have the feet sole to sole, toes pointing up and heels on the ground.

Push one person's right leg and the other's left - up, inside the arms.

Balance on the buttocks and push your foot against your partner's. Push the whole foot, toes, ball and heel together, then both slowly raise that leg.

Pull against your partner's wrists for stability, as you each straighten the leg. Now take each of your other legs up, inside the arms, pressing the second set of feet strongly against each other as you raise your other leg together.

Hold the stretch with both legs up for several seconds, then bring the first leg to be raised, slowly down **outside** the arms, feet still together. Release the second of each of your legs down **outside** the arms.

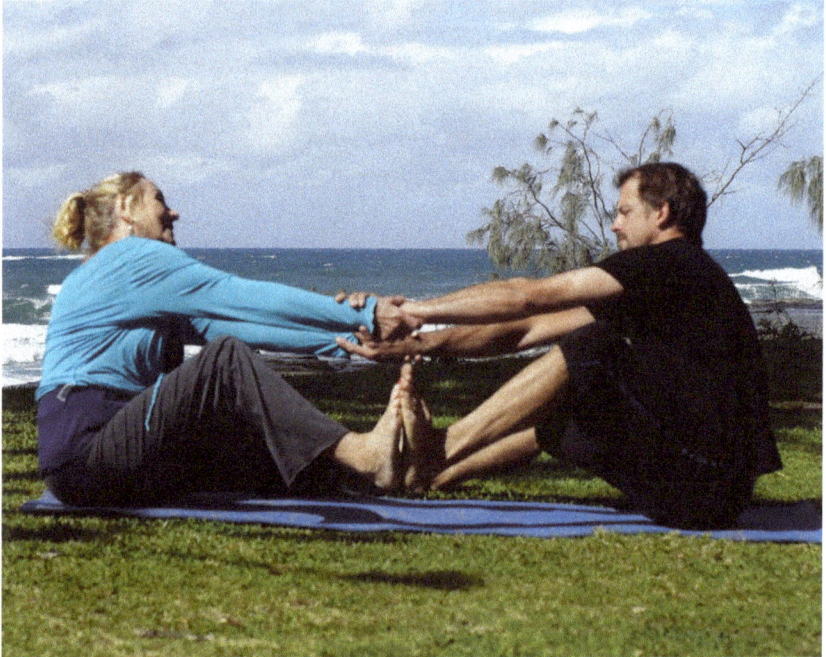

Try not to lose contact with your partner's feet and bring the legs down outside the arms. Eventually, you'll both be seated wide-legged.

Now rock around and around, one going back, one stretching forward.

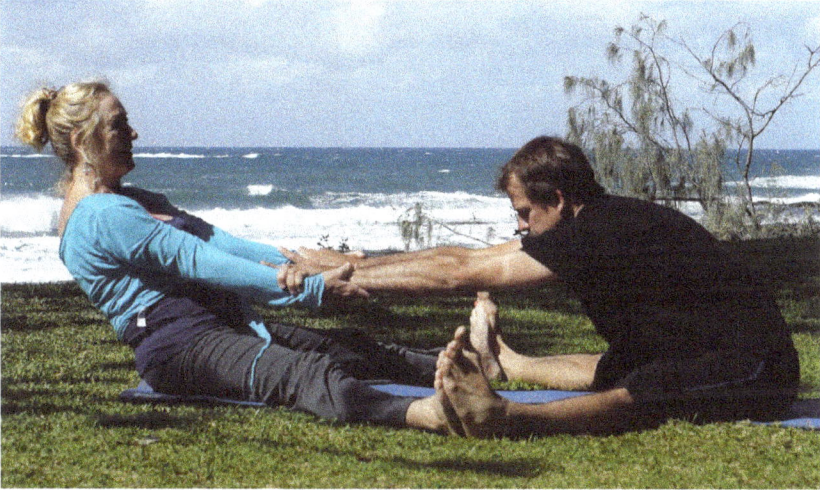

Allow one person to sway back and round, with the other coming forward as much as possible, then the forward person eases round and back, like stirring a large pot.

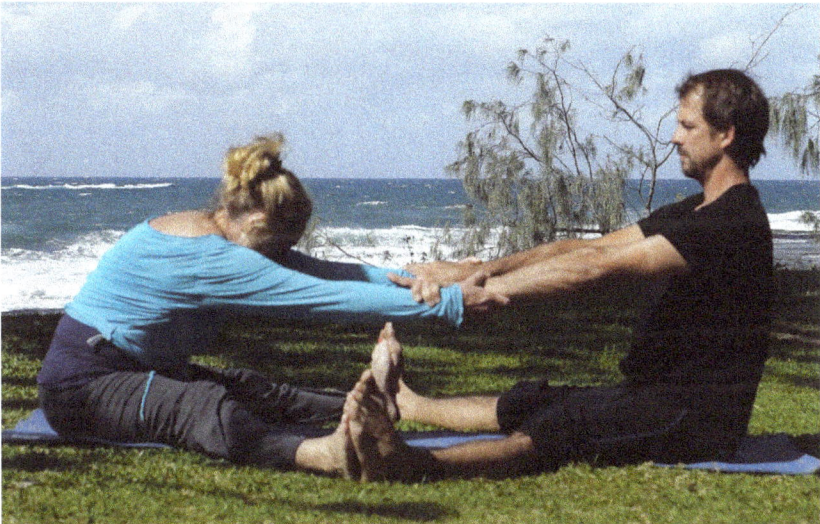

Do this both ways, reversing the direction of the 'stir'.

## BACK TO BACK SPINAL TWIST

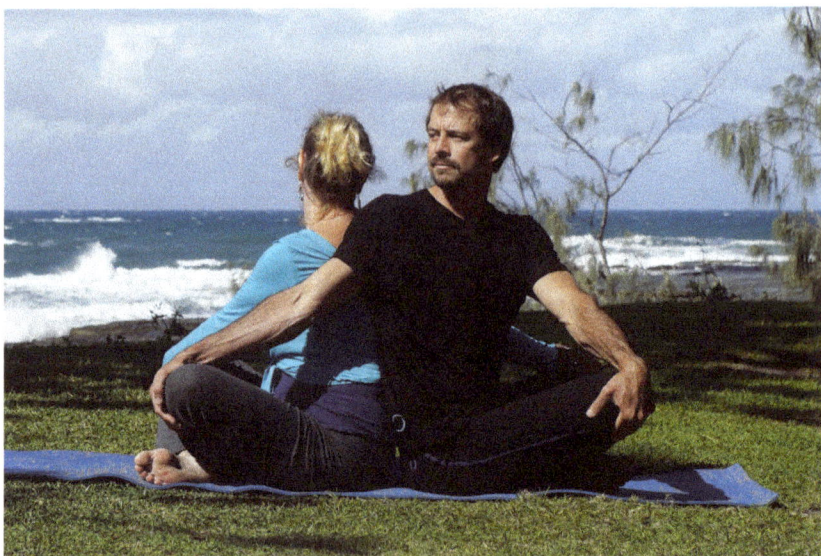

Sit back-to-back, cross-legged, backs straight and the back of the hips as close as possible. Breathe in and as you breathe out, take your right hand to your left knee and your left hand to the other person's right knee.

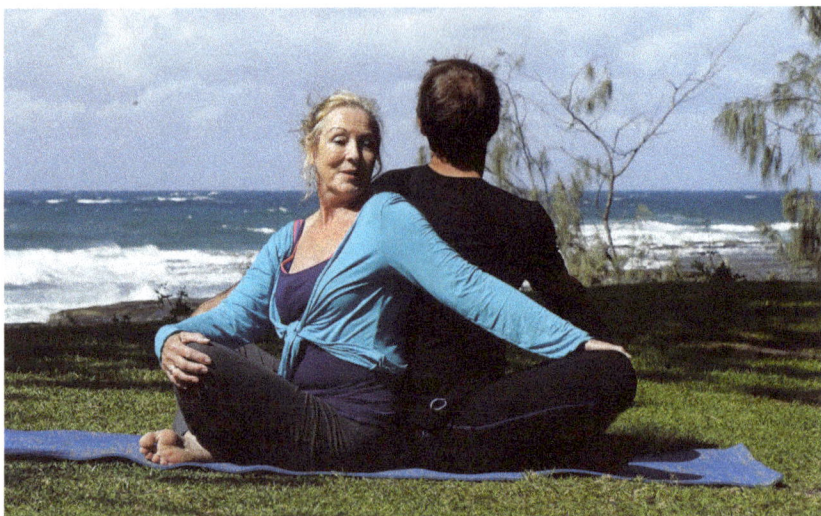

Each person does the same. Then change your arms so that on your exhalation, your left hand goes to your right knee and your right hand to their left knee. If you have long arms or are flexible, you'll be able to go further than the other person's knee such as their calf or ankle.

Depending how well you are acquainted, it may be wise to ask if it's okay to slide your arms further down their leg - as you aren't getting enough stretch just going to the knee.

To come out of the pose, simply face forward bringing your hands to your knees, then move to allow space between you.

# SECTION 6

## END LESSON POSTURES INCLUDING INVERSIONS

### CANDLE POSTURE

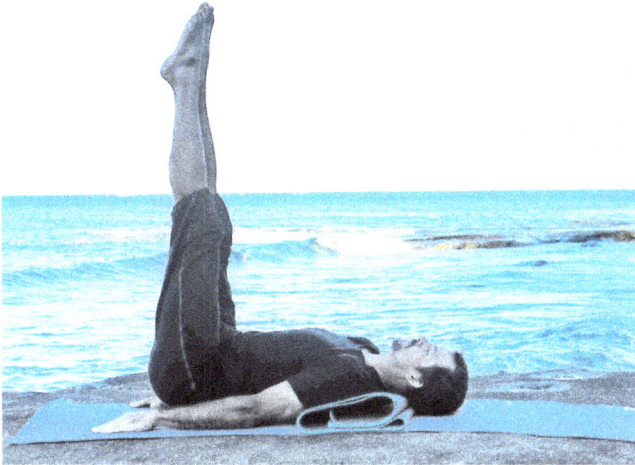

Lie on the floor then take your legs up towards the sky.

The body is on the ground except for the legs. During menstruation, this posture should be adopted rather than a shoulder-stand so as not to tip the body upside down. Inversions - upside down postures, should not be done at this time.

You can either place your hands on the floor or hold the backs of the knees.

### LEGS-UP-THE-WALL POSE - VIPARITA KARANI

If in a room, take your mat up to the wall - short edge facing the wall. Sit sideways with your hip pressed right up to the wall.

Swing your legs up the wall in a vertical position then wriggle the buttocks around so that you are facing the wall and the backs of the heels are against the wall. Allow the body to lower to the mat. There may still be a small space between your buttocks and the wall, so with your feet against the wall, wriggle closer until your buttocks, thighs and heels are against the wall.

Roll the shoulders down and back against the mat with the arms out to the sides, palms up. If this is not comfortable, have your arms out by your sides, or you may wish to stretch them out behind your head.

Remain for a minute of more. Breathe normally. To come out of this pose, bend the knees to one side and lower them to the floor.

## HALF SHOULDER STAND - ARDHA SARVANGASANA

Under normal circumstances, (not during menstruation) lie on your back. Breathe in and as you breathe out, raise your legs. Use your hands to tip the hips up.

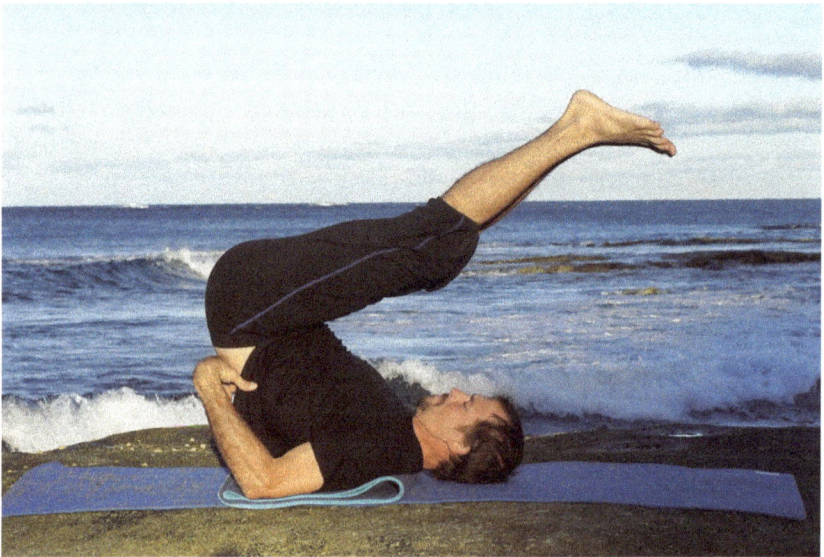

The legs will be somewhat angled towards your head initially. The weight should be on the backs of the shoulders, not the neck.

Straighten the legs.

Some students may be able to remove the hands from the hips, and with straight arms, place the palms on the calves to balance on the shoulders. If not, simply continue to support your hips with the strength of your hands.

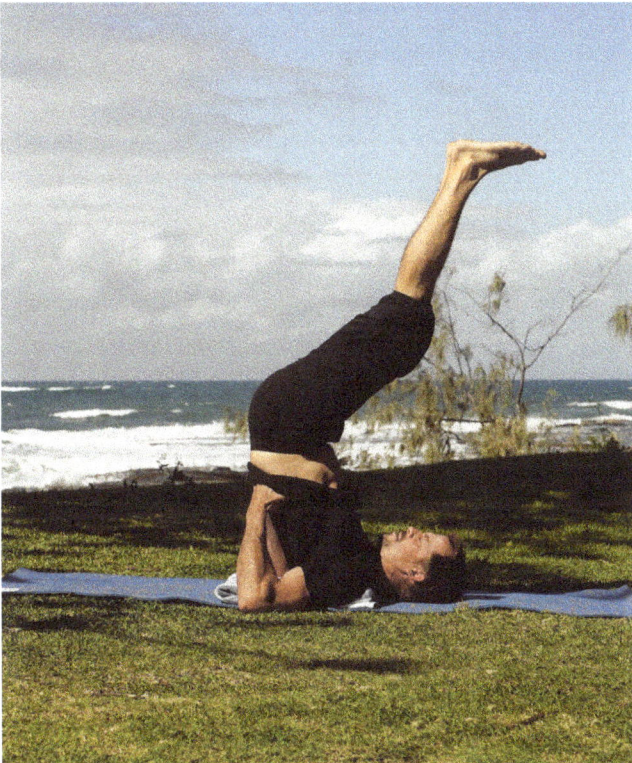

If you *will not* be going into a full shoulder stand and/or a plough posture from here, slowly roll down to the mat, vertebra by vertebra using the hands as brakes. Then proceed to perform MASTYASANA, the fish pose. (See further on in this Section).

Tipping the hips this way at the end of the class helps to rinse and rest the adrenal glands and may aid towards rectifying mid-life burn out over time.

The full shoulder stand is demonstrated below followed by the plough.

If transitioning from the half shoulder stand into the full pose, support the lower back and walk the hands a little higher up towards the bottom ribs. The elbows should be no wider than the hips. See under SARVASANGA, below.

## SHOULDER STAND - SARVANGASANA

Lie on the floor with the body in a straight line, arms by your sides. Bend the knees and bring the knees back over the chest.

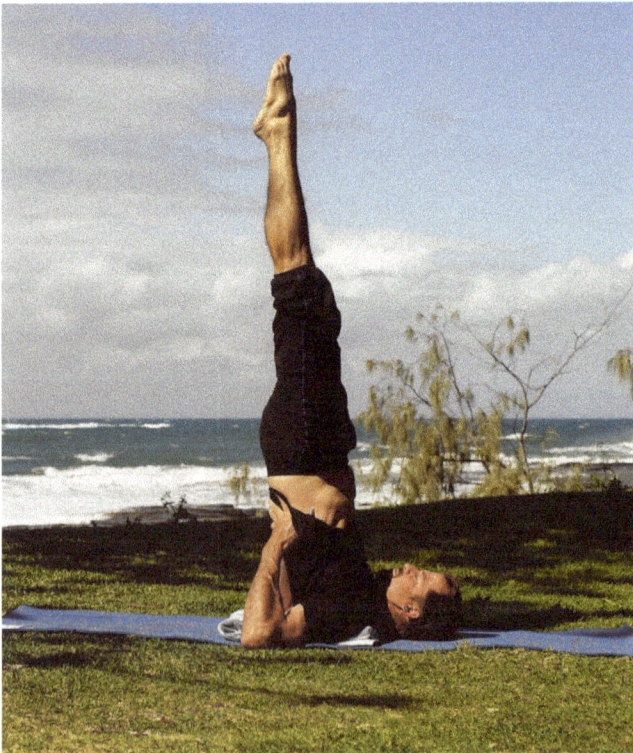

Press the elbows and upper arms into the mat. Support the middle back with the palms of the hands and thumbs. On an exhalation, raise the legs, hips, abdomen and chest higher. Come up onto the tops of the shoulders. Bring the body into a straight line.

Free breathing, in and out through the nose thereafter.

To help achieve alignment, work the hands up towards your natural arch behind the waist near to the bottom ribs and push the back of the ribs forward. Keep the elbows neatly in at the sides of the body.

Even when the legs appear straight to you, they may be slightly towards your body, with the rear-end sticking out more like a half shoulder stand - or perhaps a three-quarter shoulder stand! Tighten your abdominal muscles, continually supporting your middle back as you further straighten and align your legs with your body. Ease the chest towards your chin - *not* the other way around.

It should be noted it is difficult for many students to attain a very straight line without the use of props, for precision, such as in Iyengar Yoga. Please don't strain.

Rest assured that you will still receive a good flow of oxygenated blood to vital organs and glands.

Maintain the position for as long as comfortable; 20-30 seconds or more is recommended, if appropriate for you.

Always be mindful, and if unwell or uncomfortable, move out of a posture and relax.

To come out of the posture, angle your legs slightly towards your face, the body still elevated, but stable. Bring your hands to the mat and slowly roll down vertebra by vertebra. Use the hands as brakes on the mat.

Shoulder stand is a substitute for the headstand with almost the same benefits. It can help headache sufferers, due to stretching of the cervical spine. It sends oxygenated blood to the heart, brain and facial tissue.

Reversing the gravitational pull is refreshing for the body. However, if you feel pressure in the head, or have high blood pressure, don't maintain this posture.

## LOWERING INTO HALF SHOULDER STAND - ARDHA SARVANGASANA

From the full shoulder stand you can return to the half shoulder stand by lowering the legs towards your face. Move your hands down to support your lower back.

Stay for a few seconds, breathing normally. Maintain stability by keeping your muscles active. Finally, take your hands to the mat and ease your back down.

## LOWERING INTO THE PLOUGH - HALASANA

From shoulder-stand, continue supporting your back, exhale and take your legs over so that your feet can touch the floor behind your head as below.

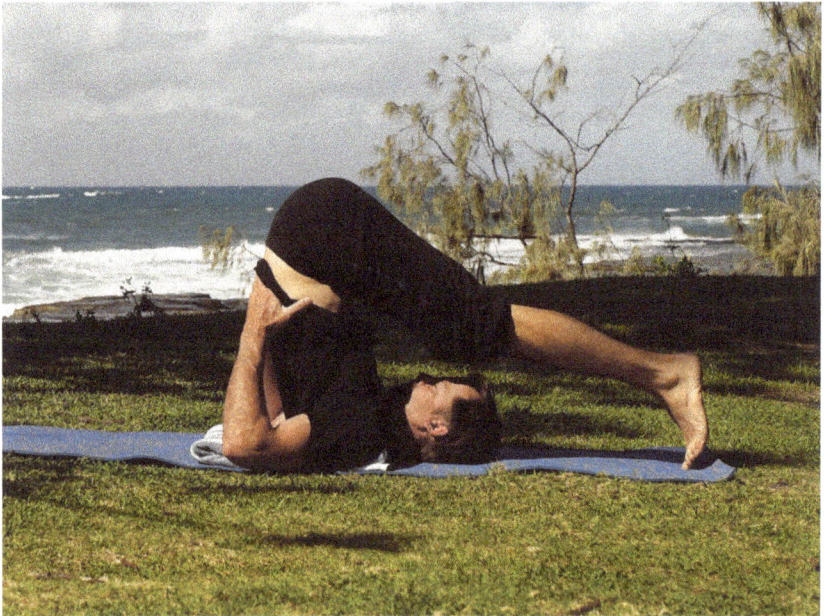

If in the plough posture, HALASANA, as depicted here, with legs extended to the floor, either rest your hands on the mat behind your body, or clasp them on the mat - again, behind the body. To exit the pose, bring the hands to the mat either side of the hips and roll down as for shoulder-stand and half shoulder-stand.

## THE PLOUGH - HALASANA

The plough is normally attempted after being in a shoulder-stand. If beginning from the mat you will approach it as you might a half shoulder stand.

Lie on your back with your hands by your sides, palms down and feet together. Keep the knees straight, inhale and as you exhale, raise the legs. On your next exhalation, bend from the hip joints and bring the legs over the body and down over your head, taking your feet to the ground behind and beyond your head.

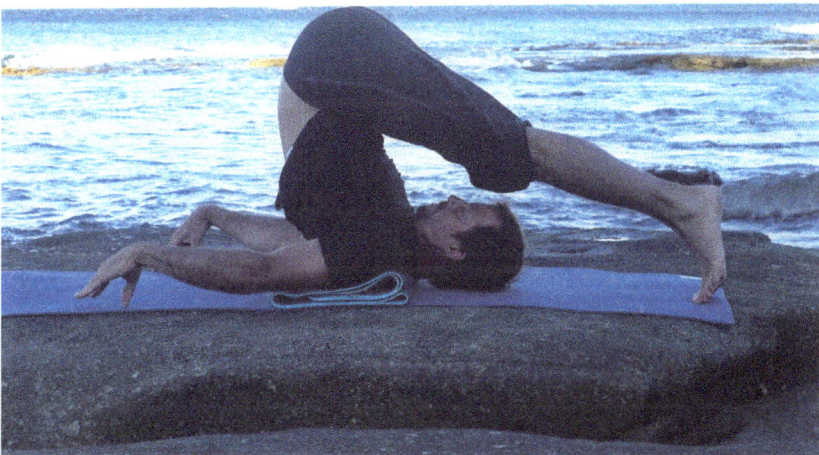

With your toes on the floor, lift the tops of the thighs and tailbone toward the sky. Draw your chin away from your sternum and soften your throat. Keep the elbows in - no wider than the shoulders.

Have your legs fully extended. Test the waters by trying one leg at a time. If they don't quite reach the floor, use a cushion, book(s), or yoga block, (previously placed).

If new to the posture keep the hands on the back. Variations for more regular practitioners: take the palms from the middle back and press them into the floor beyond your back - the opposite direction of the legs. Either have the hands palms down behind the body or clasp them together and press the arms actively down into the mat as you hold the pose.

Alternatively, if you have your feet on the floor, you can hold your ankles or toes, as shown.

Hold the posture for 20 seconds plus, as is comfortable. To exit the pose, bring your hands back to the mat then roll down onto your back, vertebra by vertebra using the hands as brakes.

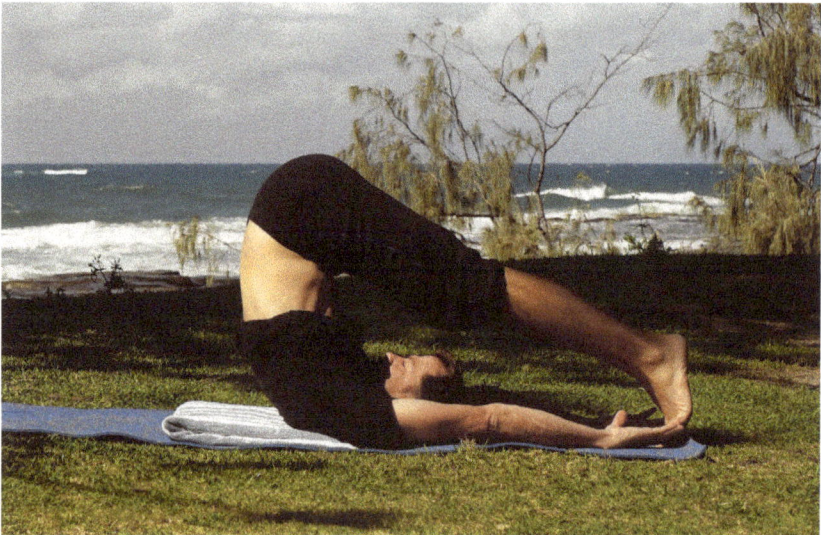

With this posture the digestive system is toned and revitalised. The entire spinal cord is stretched, spinal nerves massaged, and the nerves strengthened.

The abdominal organs, endocrine glands and reproductive organs are squeezed and toned with fresh blood circulation flowing to them. The posture helps control the metabolism and corrects hypothyroidism but it is not a good posture for goitre - an enlarged thyroid, an over-active thyroid or Graves' disease.

## THE FISH - MASTYASANA

Begin by lying on your back with your legs extended and your arms resting alongside your body, palms down.

You'll probably already be lying down on the floor after the shoulder stand, plough or half shoulder stand. This pose is a counterpose to those and should be done afterwards, your body permitting.

Press your forearms, elbows and hands into the mat by your sides. The hands and forearms can be slightly under the edge of your hips.

Breathe in and lift your shoulder blades and upper torso off the floor. Lift your chest and squeeze the shoulder blades together arching back. As you do so, tilt your head and throat backwards.

Use your elbows and forearms to continue lifting through the chest to create an arch under your upper back. Bring the crown of the head to the floor.

(If you have had a whiplash or have any other neck problem, support yourself on your arms and elbows, arching slightly back, but keeping the chin neutral).

Continue to press down through your hands and forearms. There should be very little or no weight pressing on your head. Stretch the legs and keep your thighs active. Press outward through your heels.

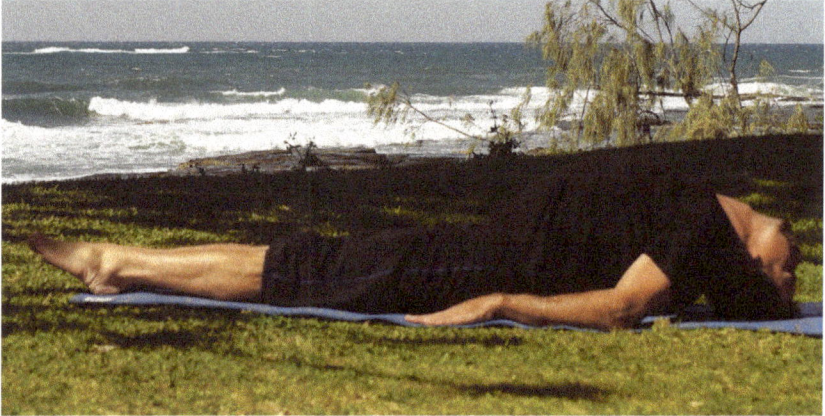

Hold the posture for approximately 10 - 20 seconds, deep breathing.

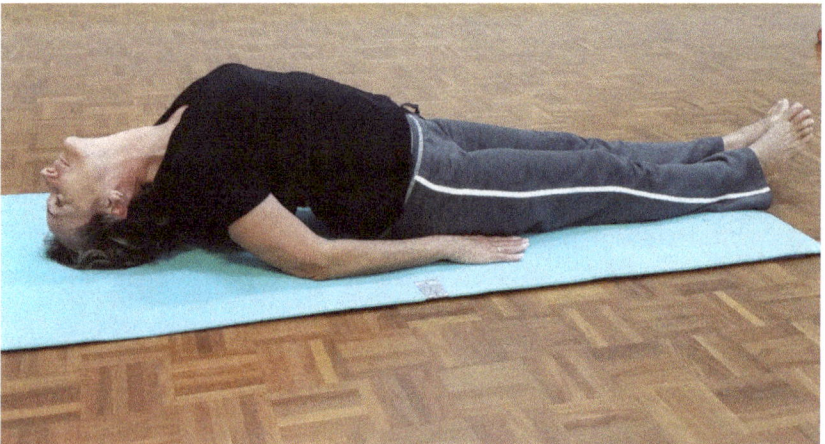

If you can maintain the arch in your back without compromising other body parts, you can bring your hands into the prayer pose over the heart centre.

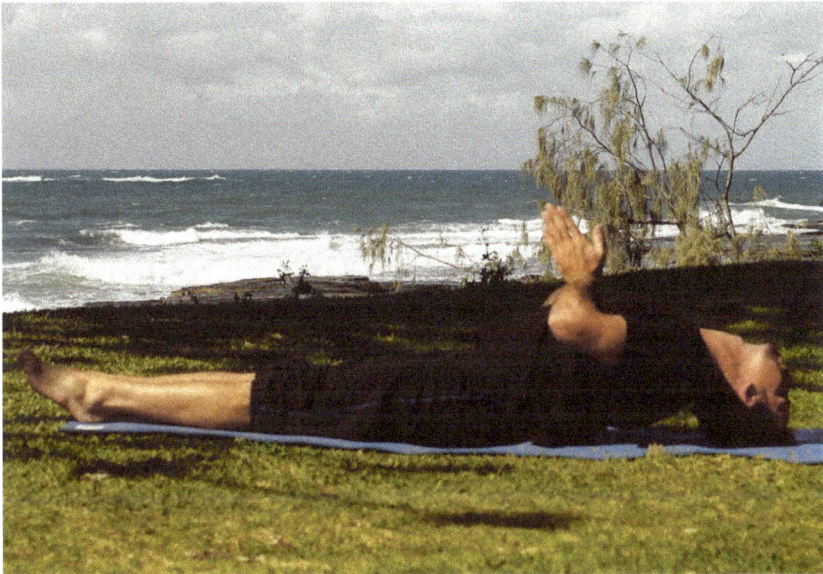

This posture is good for asthma, bronchitis and other chest conditions; it strengthens the respiratory system and relieves tension in the back and shoulders. It may correct a hunched back over time.

To release the pose, press firmly through your forearms to slightly lift your head off the floor. Exhale as you lower your torso and head to the floor.

After the posture, draw your knees into your chest then place the feet on the floor, knees bent. Take your hands behind your neck, fingers interlaced. Breathe in and stretch the neck up, breathe out, chin to chest. Repeat this two or three times to stretch and release the neck then allow the head to rest back on the mat.

## CORPSE OR RELAXATION POSE - SAVASANA

Lie on the floor with your arms and hands by your sides. Make sure the body is in a straight line. Let the feet and ankles roll out.

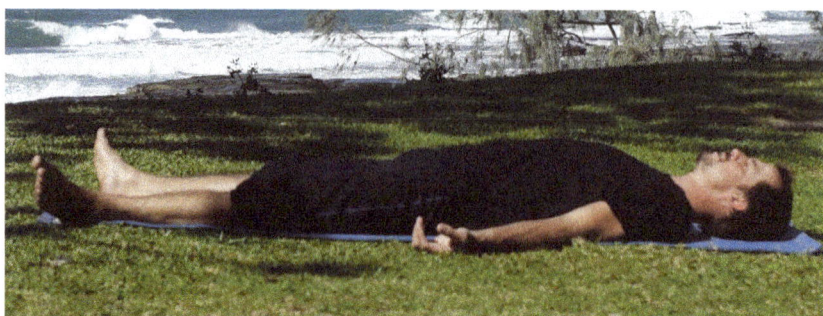

Roll the shoulders up to the ears then down and back. Allow the arms to roll outwards, palms up to the sky or ceiling. Practise deep, slow breathing in and out through the nose. As you breathe in, do so from the very bottom of the lungs, so that the whole abdominal wall moves up, first from the belly, then the waist area, into the middle chest, and finally air flows almost passively into the upper chest.

As you breathe out, the whole trunk will sink down. Be aware of that movement of the diaphragm.

As you breathe in and out through the nose, be conscious of the cool air into the nostrils, and warm air out, just above the top lip. Be aware of the skin on the cheeks either side of the nostrils and the release of tension in the face and body. SAVASANA removes fatigue from the body and quiets an agitated mind. We'll resume a longer version after pranayama and meditation.

## ROCKING UP

After yoga postures and a few minutes relaxation in the corpse posture, deep breathing, bring your knees up to your chest and hug them, then cross your ankles, hold onto your toes, and rock up into a sitting position, cross-legged.

Now you are ready for breathing exercises. After these exercises, you might resume a longer yoga relaxation and listen to a guided meditation.

# SECTION 7

## PRANAYAMA - BREATHING TECHNIQUES

---

### PRANAYAMA - BREATHING EXERCISES

When you breathe normally it is not something that you consciously think about; it just happens naturally. In pranayama, you will control the length of the breath in and out, the pause, if any, and the flow and the movement of the diaphragm.

Breathing exercises can help if you have stress, anxiety, insomnia or chronic pain. Simple slow, rhythmic breathing as described below is a good way to start.

A bird takes approximately 32 breaths a minute, a human 16 and a tortoise takes about four breaths per minute.

When we exercise we are breathing in more oxygen, which keeps the body healthy. We are not just breathing in air, but, in yogic terms, prana, or PRANIC energy - life force. It is the very essence that animates the body and makes us a living soul.

Most yoga breathing is in and out through the nose. The hairs in the nostrils filter and warm the breath on its way through to the lungs.

The nervous system depends on the breath for most of its vital energy through the nostril tract pick-up points. We lose a lot of energy by mouth breathing as we bypass these energy points.

Other vital energy we require is picked up by the nerve tips just below the skin. When we relax and breathe deeply, those 'if only' worries stored just under the skin, begin to release.

By deep breathing we oxygenate and purify the blood.

Breathing through the nose cleanses the NADIS - nerve channels, and through these, we soothe the automatic nervous system and the endocrine glands. These glands correspond to energy vortexes, or chakras, in the subtle or etheric body.

When we deep breathe, filling the lungs from the very bottom and use the whole diaphragm, we tend to respond to situations in a more relaxed manner.

To slow the breathing down short-circuits the stress response.

Additionally, as we breathe so too do the cells. In cellular respiration with deep yogic breathing, worries and past emotions locked into the cells can begin to be released.

The result of slow, deep breathing is that it activates the parasympathetic nervous system - the rest and digest engine, as opposed to the sympathetic nervous system - the survival engine. This is more fully explained in Section 9, under STRESS heading.

In short, mastery of the breath is the key to controlling the body's life force energy, so essential to good health and wellbeing.

It also allows you to access higher levels of consciousness.

Think of taking ten deep breaths in and out during moments of stress or conflict. Be conscious of your breathing.

The yoga tradition offers many time-honoured breathing techniques. Here are but a few:

## THE FULL YOGA BREATH - BREATHE TO RELAX

Once again, breathing should be slow and rhythmic, using the whole diaphragm. The *in* breath should be in three stages: abdominal, diaphragm and chest, or bottom of the lungs, middle chest/ribs, and upper chest. To begin:

Lie in the corpse posture SAVASANA or sit in a meditative pose such as SUKHASANA - the cross-legged position.

Breathing will be in and out through the nose. Close your eyes and take a few deep breaths to prepare yourself.

Firstly, take the awareness to the area of the floating ribs at the bottom of the lungs, then to the belly button and a few centimetres lower. When you breathe in, the whole abdominal wall should slowly rise from the belly as the lungs begin to expand from their bottom corners.

Place your left hand on the belly. Breathe in through your nose, into the very bottom of the lungs, firstly, so that the abdominal wall begins to rise from the lower part of the body. You should be aware of the upward motion under your hand.

Next, allow that same inhalation to continue into the middle chest and ribs, upwards and outwards, making the diaphragm expand.

Finally, expand into the upper chest - the area of the collar bones.

As you breathe out, the lungs empty and the abdominal wall goes down, towards the spine.

## KUMBHAKA (PURAKA KUMBHAKA RECHAKA)

KUMBHAKA means breath retention. There are two parts to this breath retention, one after inhalation and one after exhalation. This shouldn't be attempted if you have high blood pressure.

Sit either cross legged or on a meditation stool. You can also do this lying down. Either way, ensure the back is straight. Take a few normal breaths in and out, then breathe in fully and sharply. The breath *in* is PURAKA. Hold the breath with the lungs full. This pause is one part of KUMBHAKA - the retention of breath.

Now breathe out, which is the RECHAKA part of the exercise, then hold the breath out. Holding the breath out is the second form of breath retention also KUMBHAKA. These four parts to each breath can be practised in different ratios.

For your home practice, breathe in for the count of four, hold for the count of four, breathe out for the count of four and hold the breath *out* for the count of four, once the lungs are emptied. Never force the holding of the breath beyond comfort.

The action of PURAKA-KUMBHAKA-RECHAKA improves circulation and quiets the emotions.

## COOLING BREATH - SITALI/SHEETALI

Curl the tongue longways like a tube or pipe. Let the tongue protrude beyond the lips and inhale through your tongue-tube making a hissing sound as you suck in the air. Exhale through both nostrils. Repeat three times. SITALI cools the body.

## THE OCEAN BREATH OR VICTORIOUS BREATH - UJJAYI BREATH

Breathe in slowly through both nostrils. Relax the throat and keep the tongue back to partially close the glottis (vocal folds/muscles at the back of the mouth) then breathe out, still *through the nose* but in a stronger way than normal breathing.

The noise coming from the back of the throat will be like a muffled 'ha' sound, or the roar of the ocean. It soothes the nerves and clears the nasal passages. Repeat for three or more breaths.

## THE HUMMING BEE BREATH - BHRAHMARI

Place the index fingers or thumbs lightly into the ears. It helps to close the eyes. Inhale through both nostrils and listen to the air being drawn in.

Keep the index fingers pressed into your ears and exhale through the nose, listening to the sound of your exhalation.

Keep the mouth closed. Allow your breath out through the nose to be like a 'hum' sound.

The connection between the breath and concentration calms the mind and creates a higher awareness. It is good preparation for meditation.

## BELLOWS BREATH - BHASTRIKA

Have some tissues handy in case needed. Also, try and practise in front of a mirror. The shoulders should be relaxed and not move up and down.

This version is known as 'front bellows' as the head remains central. Other variations are not normally practised in general yoga classes. Firstly, breathe in and out deeply through the nose, filling and pushing out the lungs from the bottom as you breathe in.

Begin BHASTRIKA: exhale forcefully by contracting the abdominal muscles quickly and pumping the breath OUT, initially, one breath per second. After each out-breath, your breath *in* should be the same length. Repeat about seven times or more, breathing in and out through both nostrils. Each time you breathe out, imagine you are softly punching yourself in the stomach so that the stomach muscles contract quickly inwards.

Begin with three rounds of seven to ten out-breaths and in-breaths. Relax with normal deep breathing in between each round. Gradually increase the forceful out-breaths to two per second, and, over time, 120 breaths per round.

Bellows breath increases energy. It should either be done first thing in the morning or when you need an energy boost.

## CLEANSING OR HEAD SHINING BREATH - KAPALABHATI

This is similar to the AXE breath in Section 3. KAPALABHATI or BHASTRIKA should be the first breathing techniques of your session, followed by others.

For the standard way to perform KAPALABHATI, make sure you are sitting up straight with the head, neck and trunk of the body in alignment for this posture. Breathe in quickly; sharply.

As you exhale pull the abdominal muscles in and back towards the spine and exhale through the nose with force. After the forceful exhalation, when you release the contraction of the abdominal wall, your inhalation should be automatic, slow and passive. This breath in and out constitutes one cycle. Do seven cycles.

It purifies the blood, cleans the sinuses and respiratory passages and stimulates the digestive system.

## ALTERNATE NOSTRIL BREATHING - NADI SHODHANA PRANAYAMA

This is a simple pranayama exercise for purifying the NADIS. Closely related to the nerves, these are channels for the flow of life force energies, prana, and consciousness. They are part of an intricate web of energy within the body.

Alternate nostril breathing balances the breath in the nostrils and the flow of subtle energy within the body and the two hemispheres of the brain. It calms and centres the mind, reduces past stress and is helpful in cases of sleep apnoea, circulatory and respiratory conditions.

There are various systems. Here is a commonly used method: Sit cross-legged, or on a meditation stool with the back straight. Have the eyes half-closed or closed. Be aware of your body. Your thoughts. Have the back straight.

Rest the left hand in the lap or join the thumb and index finger and have the other fingers out straight. This is a mudra, which means gesture or sign. This particular way of joining the thumb and finger is JNANA mudra, which means wisdom or knowledge. It is also known as GYAN mudra.

Bring the right hand towards the face and rest the first two fingers at the eyebrow centre. Alternatively curl them into your palm.

Lightly close off the right nostril with the thumb and hover the ring finger above the left nostril. Exhale through the left nostril at the beginning, then breathe in through it for a few seconds. Now close the left with the ring finger, so that both nostrils are closed for an instant, then remove the thumb from your right nostril and breathe out through the right nostril. Breathe in through the right, close with the thumb, so that both nostrils are closed for an instant, remove the ring finger and breathe out left. This is one round.

And again: 1. breathe in left, 2. breathe out right, then 3. breathe in right, 4. breathe out left, (this is one full round) breathe in left again, and so on. Do seven full rounds 1 to 4. So, you are breathing IN through the same nostril you breathed OUT of. As your first breath in was on the left side, make your last breath out also on the left side, then return to normal breathing.

There are other variations of alternate nostril breathing, but this is perhaps the most commonly practised in general yoga classes. It helps balance the left and right hemispheres of the brain, harmonising the logical and emotional sides of our personality. Physiologically it cleanses the nasal passages and purifies the blood and the nerve channels: the real benefit being a relaxed body and calm mind.

The left nostril activates the nerve ending known as 'IDA' and corresponds to the parasympathetic nervous system - the more relaxed part of the autonomic nervous system. It relaxes muscles in the gastrointestinal tract and increases intestinal and gland activity. The left nostril cools the blood and relaxes the body. It corresponds to CHANDRA - the moon, and the feminine principles, such as yin and anima. Left nostril breath stimulates the **right** hemisphere of brain - the creative.

The right nostril corresponds to the nerve ending known as 'PINGALA' and corresponds to the sympathetic nervous system - the stress responder of the autonomic nervous system. Right nostril breathing gives energy and warmth - and corresponds to SURYA - the sun. It represents masculine principles such as yang and animus. The right nostril activates the **left** brain - the analytical and logical. Breathing out through the opposite nostrils calms inconsistencies within.

Of the many yogic breathing exercises, these few given will complement your home practice.

We will now look briefly at MANTRA yoga, RAJA yoga and yoga NIDRA, including stress management relaxation.

# SECTION 8

## MANTRAS

---

**MANTRA YOGA:** Union of voice and sound in repeating sounds, syllables and sacred mantras either aloud, softly or silently. This is practised for elevating and influencing the consciousness.

**NADA YOGA:** Also the yoga of sound vibration; sacred sound.

**JAPA YOGA:** Repetition in chanting mantras. It is performed prior to meditation to prepare the mind and the subtle aspects of self.

### MANTRAS - OM/AUM AND THE OM SYMBOL

You will note the Om symbol at the beginning of the book.

It consists of three curves, one semicircle, and a dot. The large bottom curve symbolises the waking state. The curve directly above it, like the top of a figure three, denotes the state of deep sleep and the curve at the side between these two curves signifies the dream state. These are our states of consciousness. The half circle, or crescent moon facing upwards, represents MAYA, illusion, which separates us from infinity or the Absolute.

This higher form of consciousness is represented by the dot.

Om is frequently called the word of glory, the transcendental 'force', the life-giver. It is the 'primordial seed' of the universe or the creative hum of the cosmic motor. It is also considered to be the root mantra or meditative seed from which all other mantras emerge.

There are also other layers of meaning. For example, the upper curve, the waking consciousness state, corresponds to humanity (and one might argue - some animals). We are self-aware and have rational consciousness.

The curve at the side represents the dream state which is said to be that of creatures: they have a dream-like consciousness.

The curve above the bottom one represents the deep sleep state, or dreamless sleep state. This is the level of consciousness of the plant kingdom and many sub-categories.

Hindu gods are also attributed to each of the three states: Brahma, Vishnu and Shiva.

Chanting om/a-u-m may be the easiest way to connect with Divinity within ourselves. When we contemplate the meaning of each of the letters, you could say we are unifying our many faceted states of consciousness, being one with all life forms and with the force that is the creator of life - the God of your perception - of your heart.

Patanjali, who wrote the Yoga Sutras, taught that when we chant this sacred syllable and contemplate the meaning of it, our consciousness becomes 'one-pointed' and prepared for meditation.

Although spelled *om*, the mantra consists of three letters, *a*, *u*, and *m* which, like the om symbol, also represents the three states of consciousness. In Sanskrit, when 'a' is followed by a 'u', it makes a long sound. The prolongation of 'm' should fade away with resonance like the chime of a distant bell.

During the intonations, Aum steps up the mind's vibratory rate. It has an effect on the pituitary and pineal glands and is transferred through the sympathetic nervous system to the other plexuses or chakras closely related to the endocrine glands.

We sail through our ordinary levels of consciousness to

the mantra's after-sound, which slowly dissolves into silence, symbolic of the transcendent state of consciousness or the Absolute.

Mantras are not unique to yoga.

In religio-magical practices throughout the world, syllables and words thought to have an influence have long been used. Early man found certain sounds were associated with divine powers and produced effects within the self, the aura, and beyond the self.

African-Americans chant 'spirituals' which often draw out the 'mmm' and the 'ah'. Many chants embody similar sounds, be they Pantheistic, Hebrew or Hare Krisna names of God, or Egyptian, Buddhist or church intonations. Mantras have power to create or enhance.

Sanskrit mantras are said to have distinct potency and power. There are many 'seed' mantras such as Krim, Shrim, Hrim, Dum, Hum, Gum, Huam, Glaum, Gam, Kshraum, Strim, Aim and others.

Seed mantras mean they are used along with other words for a certain purpose or outcome.

Lam, Vam, Ram, Yam, Ham and Om are used in connection with the chakras:

Root or base chakra - Lam;
Sacral - Vam;
Solar plexus - Ram;
Heart - Yam;
Throat - Ham;
Third eye - Om, (sometimes Ksham or Kshraum, is used);
Crown - Om.

Om Mani Padme Hum is popular in Tibetan culture to bring about compassion.

To keep things simple for your home practice *Om/Aum* is easy to remember and universal. It can precede meditation or relaxation.

There is a source at the end of the book for those interested in pursuing mantras.

# SECTION 9

## MEDITATION AND RELAXATION

---

## MEDITATION

RAJA YOGA: Refining the mind. A process of meditation - being ruler of the mind.

YANTRA YOGA: Where mantra yoga influences the consciousness through sound, yantra yoga uses sight for the same purpose. Mandalas, inspiring pictures or symbols can be used, as can something visualised by the mind.

Things you may need to organise first:

Ensure you take care of any bodily needs first, such as having a few sips of water. It's no good to be thinking about how uncomfortable you are during meditation, rather than achieving profound peace through it.

Listed below are ideas for 'props' to have handy prior to sitting in meditation:

A mediation stool or cushion.

If you would like to focus your attention on an object, bring it into the space in front of your eye level or at easy gazing distance. This may be a candle, flower - such as a rose and its petals, a mandala, a labyrinth or other sacred shape, symbol or picture.

If outside, you might choose to gaze at a leaf or the sunlight through the trees.

If near the ocean, on the line between ocean and sky - that fine white haze which hovers between the two.

Alternatively, you might meditate on your third eye at the centre of the forehead, or on the heart centre.

Meditation is to create a calm, still, peaceful mind. It is the suspension of everyday thought. It seeks to blend with universal consciousness.

The master gland, the pituitary gland, is in the centre of the head. Further back is the lesser known gland, the pineal. This is thought to be the gland which translates subconscious impressions into understandable ideas for our conscious mind to understand.

When the mind is still, we are more aware of higher consciousness. Meditation on the third eye is the gateway to this higher realm of consciousness.

If you have a very busy mind, you may find concentrating on an object, such as a mandala, symbol, picture or flower, rather than the third eye, to be more useful.

Alternatively, meditate on a candle flame (Please make sure your candle is safe, preferably contained and can't topple over).

Choose a theme that this symbol might help achieve, such as peace, world peace, universal love, compassion, heart-centredness, reintegration with your divinity, healing on all levels of being, world healing and so on.

When you have what you need, physically and in the mind, sit on a meditation stool, cross-legged or even on a straight-backed chair if yoga methods are not comfortable for you.

Ensure the spine is straight. Squeeze in the dorsal muscles, ease the shoulder blades in, straighten to the crown of the head and relax the shoulders.

Begin with breathing exercises which will include seven rounds of NADI SHODHANA, alternate nostril breathing. Focus on your chosen 'prop'. Let us say it is a picture of the OM symbol.

Your theme might then be *peace and compassion between all living systems*, and with divinity. As above, so below, so to speak.

Continue with this theme. Now to silencing the busy mind in order to focus ready for meditation.

## PRATYHARA - Withdrawal of the Senses

After the restraints and observances (YAMA and NIYAMA) in daily life and within your yoga practice of ASANAS and PRANAYAMA, comes PRATYHARA, withdrawal of the senses.

PRATYHARA is the bridge between the outer or profane world and the sacred or inner world of yoga and the further stages of meditation.

Chanting isn't necessarily part of PRATYHARA, but can work in tandem with it. Try chanting in your mind, then softly, then louder. If you have your own sacred space, chant several A-U-Ms aloud. Focus on the vibration of the sound even if the sound is only in your mind.

Withdraw your senses from the outer world of distractions. Go within. Be aware of the third eye centre or the heart centre.

Let go of everyday thoughts. Let thoughts come in and go out. Observe them as they float through your stream of consciousness without giving them time and energy. Don't interact with them.

Imagine thoughts like sparks of light in, and out, floating away. Allow your mind to clear. Aim to be master of your thoughts - not let them be master of you.

Train your mind to return from outer distraction to your inner world - the spark of consciousness that you are.

## DHARANA - Concentration

After withdrawing the senses as above, this step, DHARANA, is about holding the attention, being present. It is where you will concentrate and focus on an object.

This can be to concentrate on a physical object, or it can also be the third eye or heart centre. If so, you could visualise a violet dot at the centre of your forehead, or a pink haze at the heart centre.

Your object can be simply being aware of your breath in, and your breath out. If so you might attribute the OM mantra to each inhalation and exhalation. Your point of focus could also be an actual repetitive chant of a mantra.

Close the eyes or half-close them so that you are vaguely aware of the light and your chosen symbol, real or imagined. Concentrate on your symbol and what it represents to you (the spiritual theme). Focus on it. Allow yourself to be absorbed by the symbol.

## DHYANA - Meditation

Through a steady and continuous focus towards this chosen thing, a state of meditation can be achieved for a period of time - however brief.

There comes an awareness that is different from every-day reality. This is a state of *being*, rather than doing. Then, as you blend into oneness with the universe, another level of reality occurs - bliss.

## SAMADHI - Oneness/super-consciousness/ecstasy

This is when you experience the consciousness that you are (as opposed to the body/mind/emotions) and are at one with the greater whole. It is an 'attuning' with the universe and beyond. It can also be described as an ecstatic calm. Remain for 10 - 20 minutes.

You will have heard of other meditative experiences through the practice of KUNDALINI YOGA.

LAYA YOGA/ KUNDALINI YOGA/ KRIYA YOGA are about the arousal of the force which is considered psychic nerve energy and/or the awakening of the kundalini energy, not mentioned in this book, as they should be undertaken under the supervision of a qualified teacher. TANTRA YOGA also falls into this category.

**Kundalini awakening** is an electrophysiological occurr-ence in tandem with a mystical awakening. Unsupervised, practitioners could have ill effects.

Suffice to say, if you are being mindful of your actions, observing the self and correcting inconsistencies, practising hatha yoga with breathing exercises, some meditation and relaxation, you will slowly, over time, activate a higher level of awareness, increase wellbeing and release some emotional blocks.

## RELAXATION

YOGA NIDRA: Relaxation or psychic sleep

Lie down on the mat and make sure your body is in a straight line. If you don't have a relaxation CD/ guided meditation, try the following:

Relax the feet and allow the ankles to roll outwards. Roll the shoulders up to the ears then outward and down. Let the arms fall out, palms facing the ceiling. Begin deep breathing in and out through the nose. Firstly, be aware of the toes and the feet. Tighten the feet, the calves, thighs and buttocks, then release, let go.

Press the middle back into the mat, then let go, and allow your back to resume its natural curve. Breathe in and take the top tips of the shoulders to the mat, arching slightly, then relax the back.

Turn your head to the left and to the right, then back again. Let the hips open and relax. Be aware of cool breath into the nose, and warm air out, just above the top lip. Be aware of the diaphragm rising and falling with each breath.

Imagine slipping through a rainbow of colour, one colour at a time starting with warm reds and pinks as you feel the body tighten, release and relax. With each breath out, imagine letting go of physical heaviness.

As you slip from pinks into warm orange, let go of emotional concerns and discord. With each breath out, let go of everyday thoughts. Stop thinking about what you have to do and what you haven't done. Let it go, for now, and imagine thoughts going on a sunbeam of golden yellow.

Feeling lighter, let your golden yellow merge into the green of nature and imagine floating through a valley, seeing the grass, trees and leaves - the many shades of green. In your minds-eye, look up between branches into blue. Allow your blue to change from a noon-day blue sky to a night sky of indigo then violet skies with planets and stars. You are as a spark of light, a spark of consciousness, merging back into the greater whole, like a star in the sky or a drop of dew in the ocean.

Continue for as long as peace prevails or is appropriate then blink your eyes, take a few steadying breaths and relax.

This relaxation can be done in much more depth by going through each body part centimetre by centimetre, each toe, each joint from the soft pads of the toes to the crown of the head. In this way you are present, yet rested.

## STRESS

You need a certain amount of stress or you wouldn't get out of bed in the morning. There are certain changes in life, which are stressful to most people.

These main stresses in modern life are: death, (someone else's) at the top of the list, break-up, injury and illness. Buying a house or marriage is about half-way on the stress scale and even going on holiday is about a quarter of the way up the scale. Naturally there are stresses connected with careers, business and finance as well as family and friend discord and so on, all of which take their place on the scale.

We have a biochemical response to stress. Impulses surge to the adrenal glands - part of the endocrine nervous system. This increases the breathing, heartrate, alertness and even muscle response. We are then 'on edge' - ready for action. Ultimately, the body's metabolism speeds up and we become enmeshed in the 'fight or flight' syndrome - ready to fight the tiger in the jungle, but if there's no danger, no tiger, then it is an 'over-the-top' reaction and not good for us.

Yoga helps create balance and calmness when faced with stress by working on the autonomic nervous system and the endocrine glands. The autonomic nervous system, or endocrine system as it is also known, is a selection of glands: the pituitary, pineal, hypothalamus, thyroid, parathyroid, adrenals, pancreas, and ovaries/testes which pass their hormones directly into the blood stream.

Whereas our spinal or central nervous system and brain use electrical impulses and are responsible for most functions of the body, mind, and our objective and subjective states of consciousness, the autonomic nervous system uses hormones to communicate super sensory impressions to plexuses and glands. The hormones effect changes in our body such as emotions, cognitive responses and even energy.

The autonomic nervous system has two strands, firstly, the sympathetic nervous system, mentioned earlier, which is activated in response to stress. Besides the physiological aspects, the sympathetic nervous system is associated with the subconscious mind. The subconscious influences the mind. Our conscious mind and thoughts influence our subconscious. It's a two-way street.

Secondly, the parasympathetic nervous system: This is involved in routine activities. The parasympathetic nervous system is associated with higher consciousness, in charge of our unconscious state where thought isn't involved. It is the more restful strand of the autonomic nervous system.

Postures massage the endocrine glands. Deep breathing sets up a connection between the subtle and dense bodies to bring about harmony and relieve tiredness and stress.

Meditation and meditative relaxation techniques decrease oxygen consumption, the heart and respiratory rates and the blood pressure. These decreases are the opposite of the physiological changes which take place during the stress response. Therefore, meditation is ideal for the heart, breath, body, and blood pressure; in short for physical, mental and emotional health.

Meditation also increases the alpha, theta and delta brain wave intensity.

**ALPHA:** Relaxed state of mind. Passivity. Relaxation. Meditation. Sometimes achieved through intense creativity such as art.

**BETA:** The wakeful state

**THETA:** Sleep. Very deep meditation. Ecstasy.

**DELTA:** Deep dreamless sleep.

Alpha and theta states can be achieved during meditation and relaxation.

The delta state is best saved until after you have finished your meditation practice. Meditation will aid a good peaceful sleep.

Meditation takes you from the space you are in to an alternative reality - to 'stand back' from a situation.

In addition to soothing the autonomic nervous system, more oxygen and life force energy - prana, comes into the body, through the postures, relaxation and deep breathing.

Through the corridors of time, yoga has taught the body-mind-soul connection.

After you return to the secular aspects of life, make each moment sacred by being present and mindful of your body, thoughts, words, deeds and actions.

You read at the beginning of the book that before yoga actions, breathing and so on, there was YAMA at the top of the list on page two, and depicted as the base of the pyramid on page five. Yama was about being present, being honest, kind in thoughts, words, deeds and so on: non-injury to self or others. The word used was Ahimsa. It means non-injury in thought, word or deed.

# SECTION 10

## FOOD FOR THOUGHT

### DIET

We cannot close without mentioning how the 'deed' part of Ahimsa relates to diet. It means non-injury to living being, thus choosing cruelty-free food, foods with life-force from the earth. The yoga diet is vegetarian, and these days, for many, vegan.

The physical component of food is but the outer tantaliser. We must bear in mind there is both an emotional and a spiritual part of food. The food feeds our emotional and our spiritual beings.

Yoga nutrition means eating natural food, which has 'prana' or life force such as pervades living organic products. Chemicals and colouring don't fall into this category, nor do starch, flour and sugars. Yoga divides food thus: There are three food qualities, or GUNAS, affecting our personalities:

**TAMAS GUNA (Tamasic):** These are heavy, lead-like, decaying and fermented products, such as meat, alcohol, intoxicants, drugs, tobacco, processed and chemically treated foods and additives. Contaminated food, food that is hard to digest, overeating and food prepared without good energy by the person handling it, are also considered tamasic. Such foods are negative, self-destructive and can cause inertia. The prana, or life force, is withdrawn from tamasic foods so they do not benefit mind or body.

**RAJAS GUNA (Rajasic):** Hot and spicy, salty, bitter and sour such as piquant spices, strong herbs or stimulants. Coffee, tea, and 'feel good' foods containing salt, spices and sugar, including chocolate and fried foods, are also rajasic.

These are active, passionate and emotional foods. They give energy, but it burns out quickly. Activities that require movement are stimulated by rajasic foods. However, while it promotes motivation, energy and action, too much rajasic food overexcites the body and causes strong emotionally charged qualities, passions and responses. It makes the mind restless and upsets the mind-body equilibrium.

**SATTVA GUNA (Sattvic):** Legumes - beans and lentils, grains, seasonal organic fruit and vegetables, nuts and seeds, plant-based oils, honey and cinnamon. Some spices such as turmeric, coriander and basil fall into this category. The energy from sattvic food is light and gives vitality. Being fresh from the ground or tree, sattvic food has life force - prana, because plants consume sunlight, air and water. The yoga diet is sattvic.

You may argue that carrots scream when pulled from the ground, and indeed their response to stimuli has been registered. Plant and vegetable life respond to music and environment, so they will 'register' being pulled out of the ground. However, they live in sleeping consciousness as depicted in the Om symbol. They do not have an intricate brain and a central nervous system. Therefore, as far as we know, their response to being uprooted isn't the same as pain experienced by creatures.

There are people uncomfortable with the concept of ripping food out of the earth. They choose to only eat that which drops from the trees and are fruitarian.

For explaining the yoga diet, the concept of ahimsa relates more to not harming our walking, swimming, flying, slithering or other breathing socialising beings, than it does to interfering with the sleeping consciousness of a root vegetable.

When we eat fruit or vegetables, we don't say we are going out to the garden to kill a carrot or a tomato. We pick it. We pick, gather or harvest fruit and vegetables like we harvest grain or rice.

**Dairy:** The yoga diet has a history of including dairy. Hindus have long revered their cows as sacred. They didn't consume them. Dairy Farms in India only had a small number of cows. Dairy products were always part of the sattvic diet.

These days, whatever country it is, the way we treat milk and egg producing entities makes dairy products tamasic, not sattvic, because of the horrors the animal endures during intensive farming, transportation and at the end of its life.

**Eggs:** Even if you buy free range eggs, when the mother chickens were babies, there were also baby boy chickens born. Lots of them. Where are they? Virtually all the boy chickens, who have no commercial value, are gassed or disposed of in a less favourable way, at birth.

Today, the dairy industry we know throughout most of the world, keeps cows pregnant year after year so that when lactating after having given birth, we can acquire their milk.

Their babies, the calves, will never enjoy their mother's milk. Both male and female calves are taken away soon after birth and fed on a commercial, watery milk substitute.

Many female calves will replace worn out older cows, and when mature, will have a life like their mothers: incarcerated and pregnant, followed by full udders and their babies taken away a few days after birth.

Some females will be sent to slaughter and almost all male calves, known as bobby calves, are slaughtered, unless they are kept for veal (young flesh) and killed later. Veal calves are slaughtered anytime up to eighteen weeks of age, depending on the type of veal required. Having no commercial value, bobby calves don't even receive the same basic care as female calves, and calves kept for veal, before being sent to slaughter.

A growing number of people see the mother and baby separation as being as cruel as the killing floor of the meat industry. These days the vegetarian stance of many, including yoga practitioners, is broadening to embrace veganism.

Early humanity didn't know better; they hunted to survive, as well as forage for plant food. Then about 10,000-12,000 years ago, we started to grow food and keep animals for our convenience.

Later, in the mid-1800s, Charles Darwin's theories of evolution and social adaptation, amid group struggle and competition, was the key to survival. Animals and humans existed as fruits of a single 'tree' and since humans were the most highly 'evolved' they were only performing their evolutionary role by metabolising as much protein from other creatures as possible.

Like animals we have become creatures of survival. We are so busy keeping our place in the world we have little time to think about what we consume, who has suffered as a result, and if it is doing us, the planet, or other nations any good in the long term.

We no longer need to kill animals to survive and as human consciousness evolves, many choose other diets.

However, parts of the world continue to breed cloven-footed beasts and other species, to slaughter. We refer to these beings as livestock. Stock is an accounting term, hence we mean 'living consumables', walking, breathing, socialising mortals that can be killed and utilised.

## ECOLOGICAL CONSEQUENCES

By breeding animals in such large quantities, we are suffering the ecological consequences. Flatulence and burping from the world's billion plus domestic grazing animals is playing a role in climate change. By farming livestock - cattle, sheep, goats, pigs and chickens, the world contributes almost 6 billion tonnes of greenhouse gases - which includes carbon dioxide, methane, and nitrous oxide from feed production, into the atmosphere each year.

These gases, along with land clearing, water resources

and soil acidity are just some of the problems having a significant environmental impact by continuing such large-scale animal farming.

In summary: What you put on your plate has an impact on the environment. Meat and dairy are more resource intensive than plant-based foods.

## HUMAN TO HUMAN COOPERATION

Plant protein could feed more people:

The land grabbing avarice that spawned the cattle industry from around the 1700s has transformed countries, particularly the American mid-west, Argentina and Australia, into gigantic cattle breeding grounds.

Besides ecological consequences, lands used for beef cattle or to grow sorghum feed for the cattle, rather than native crops, have left other parts of the world hungry.

The animal agriculture industry that pervades western culture takes up nearly 60% of our planetary land mass if we include the growing of feed for cattle. Grazing land is over 26%. A further third of the arable land is used for the cultivation of livestock feed crops.

Back in the 1970s, Ethicist Peter Singer argued that an acre of land could be used to grow a high-protein plant food like beans and the yield would be 300-500 pounds. Plant protein was fed to animals, then the animals were killed for food, yielding 45-55 pounds from the same acre.

Since the 1960s livestock protein production has approximately tripled. Instead of consuming a certain percentage of food directly from the land, we have transferred more of our direct consumption of plant foods into *growing feed* for livestock. Three quarters of the world's land mass used for animal agriculture produces about only about 37% of protein.

An acre of cereal produces five times more protein than

an acre used for animal protein production. Plant-based agriculture, such as legumes, yields ten times more protein. Water used to produce animal products ranges from a third more, to excessively more than water needed to produce soy milk and vegetarian produce.

There would be enough cropland to feed 9 billion people in 2050 - *if* the 40 percent of all crops produced today *for feeding animals* were used for growing produce for human consumption.

Since we could feed more people with plant protein, it would embrace human to human cooperation in addition to the obvious benefits to animals and the earth.

## FOUR FOOTED FEASTS - HEALTH

Living atop the protein ladder is precarious for some. There are health related problems such as heart attack, cancer and diabetes. These are all diseases of affluence due in a large part to our diet. The poor, almost a billion, languish worldwide without enough food and two billion don't have access to safe drinking water. They teeter on the brink of despair, hoping to climb the protein ladder, while the western world devours four-footed feasts to their detriment.

Plant food receives the sun's energy and light directly, but only 10% of the sun's energy, captivated by photosynthesis to produce plant tissue, is converted to energy in the tissue of herbivores. Of that, only 10% again reaches the tissue of carnivores. The amount of energy decreases every step in the food chain. When humans eat meat, they are not directly linked to the sunlight and energy of the plant. Hence it is more efficient for us to follow Ahimsa and eat cereals, fruit, and vegetables as we are consuming foods with light, life force and energy as mentioned in the discussion of yogic sattvic foods.

Additionally, the adrenaline released when animals are

fearful and stressed before slaughter uses up glycogen, which would be converted into lactic acid after death, and would keep the meat tender. Without it, flesh goes off more rapidly. It will be tough and the level of acidity likely to be high.

The adrenaline overload of the terrified animal is taken into the body along with hormones, toxic chemicals and genetic tampering used to artificially stimulate growth for increased yield.

## THOUGHT FORMS

As stated at the beginning of the book, thoughts are real things.

Through time, people sensitive to psychic vibrations maintain that these energy forms, or thought patterns, hover around and emanate from a person or creature.

Around and above positive, good people, esoteric, humane and joyous venues, the energy or thought patterns are peaceful.

Above abattoirs, as in battlefields, there are energy globules put out by animals who are about to be killed, or who have been recently killed. These thought forms are troubled and negative.

Just as a masseur can pick up negative vibrations from massaging a client, it could be argued that when eating meat, we take on the stress vibrations of the dead animal - within the product being eaten. (Hence the saying, 'You are what you eat').

## PURIFYING

Certain esoteric organisations of east and west suggest that vegetarianism or better still, veganism, may be better for health and for some days prior to a special meditation.

The priests and priestesses of ancient times (including

Jesus) fasted before meditating.

A sensible inclination towards vegetarianism, combining the right food groups and trying new vegetarian or vegan taste sensations, if only five out of seven days, may lighten our bodies and aid meditations and insights.

## ETHICAL CONSIDERATIONS

## CLOSENESS TO OTHERS

About 99% of human genes are identical to corresponding ones in chimpanzees. We are kin to them and other organisms, particularly the bonobo, also known as pygmy chimpanzee.

We are also apart from the gorilla, orangutan, other apes and monkeys, and indeed other animals, by a matter of degrees. Yet, until recently, a large percentage of humanity have given less value to the interests of nonhuman animals. Now, the minority voices are being joined by the masses. We see that by condoning intensive farming, live export transportation, animal experimentation and all other facets of animal dominion which cause suffering, we are not being the best we can be.

## SLAVERY

The live animal export trade has been compared with that of slavery. Human slavery is considered the height of exploitation. The only difference is that instead of using humans, we are submitting animals, the creatures with whom we share such close DNA, to the control of various others and treating them as property, hence while animal exploitation continues, we are speciesist - but changes are in the air.

## SPECIESISM

Sexist and racist behaviour have blazed the trail of history, but until now little thought has been given to the human view towards other sentient beings.

It is the same basic tenet not to consider animals as not to consider minority groups or indigenous cultures. Animals talk a different language - dance to the sound of a different drum, but we are all one.

## THE DARK NIGHT TO THE LIGHT
The world has millions of cloven-footed beasts putting out CO2 one end and methane the other. He or she has suffered, has been artificially inseminated or castrated, is full of hormones, some even genetically altered. He or she is treated as a nameless item of stock, consumed without honour.

Ahimsa proposes that we extend altruism to all creatures. Irrespective of environmental, global food and health issues, eating fellow non-human animals and keeping them in cramped conditions is not good for their evolution. Animals participate in the Divine Plan. It could be argued they are humans in the making.

## BACK TO BASICS
Remember the building blocks where we began, at the beginning of this book – the pyramid beginning with YAMA, NIYAMA, ASANA, PRANAYAMA and so-on?

Through these steps, yoga can be present in our daily lives, taking care of our whole being: the spiritual, intellectual, emotional, psychic and the physical - including that which is consumed.

We need to be mindful, the ancient Buddhist and Hindu concept of being present and aware. Study the different facets of YAMA and NIYAMA. See if you can bring your awareness into your thoughts, words and actions, including awareness when performing yoga asanas. Be aware of the movement and the sensation within your body, and enjoy your home practice - keeping it up.

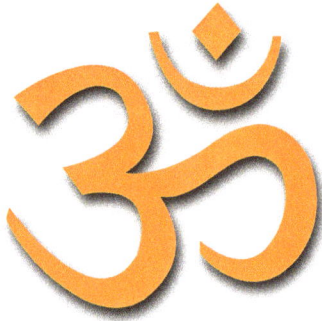

# Bibliography

Anonymous by request I.C. 2018, An abattoir worker, Queensland.

Ashley-Farrand, T. 1999, *Healing Mantras*, Ballantine Books, a division of Random House Publishing Group, New York.

*Atlas of Anatomy*, 2005, (2003) Giunti Editorial Group, Florence.

Besant, A and Leadbeater C.W. 1961, (1901) *Thought Forms*, The Theosophical Publishing House, Adyar.

International Society for Krisna Consciousness, 1997, *Chant and Be Happy: The Power of Mantra Meditation*, The Bhaktivedanta Book Trust, LA.

Batmanghelidj, F. 1995 (1992), *Your Body Cries for Water*. Global Health Solutions, VA, USA.

Bloom, W. 2011 (2001), *The Endorphin Effect*, Piatkus Books, Little Brown Book Group, London.

Bronowski, J. 1973, *The Ascent of Man*, Sir Joseph Causton & Sons, London.

Capra, F. 1996, *The Web of Life*, Anchor, division of Bantam Doubleday Bell, New York.

Cameron, J and S.A. 2017, 'Animal agriculture is choking the Earth and making us sick. We must act now,' *The Guardian*, Australian edition, 4 December.

Carrington, D. 2018, 'Huge reduction in meat-eating 'essential' to avoid climate breakdown', *The Guardian*, Australian edition, 10 October.

Darwin, C. 1968 (1859), *The Origin of Species*, Penguin, London.

Dennett, D.C. 1995, *Darwin's Dangerous Idea: Evolution and the meanings of life*, Simon & Schushter, New York.

Delforce, C. 2018, *Dominion*, film documentary, Australia.

Dupont, P. 2009, *The Endocrine Glands, and Your Health*, The Rosicrucian Order AMORC Sydney (Originally published in French as Les Grandes Endocrines et Notre, Disffusion Rosicrucienne, Chateau d'omonville. Le Tremblay).

*Faunalytics*, 2017, 'Farming Animals Vs. Farming Plants - A Comparison' Olympia, 4 July.

Fisher, A. 2013, 'Can live export ever be humane?' *The Conversation*, 3 November, viewed 9 June, 2018, <https://theconversation.com/live-animal-export-problems-begin-in-our-own-paddock

Gossard, M. A. 2003, 'The Social and Structural Influences of Meat Consumption' in *Research in Human Ecology*, Washington State University, Pullman.

Hewitt, J. 1987 (1977), *The Complete Yoga Book*, Century Hutchinson, London.

International Yoga Teachers Association (IYTA) 1984, *Handbook of Traditional Asanas*, Sydney.

Iyengar, B.K.S. 1976 (1968), *Light on Yoga*, Unwin Paperbacks, London.

Iyengar, B.K.S. 2014 (2001), *Yoga: The Path to Holistic Health*, Dorling Kindersley, Penguin-Random House, London.

Iyengar, B.K.S. 1993, *Light on Pranayama*, Harper Collins, India.

Jordanova, L. J. 1984, *Lamarck*, Oxford University Press, Oxford.

Kaminoff, L. 2007, *Yoga Anatomy*, Human Kinetics, USA.

McEwan, G 2011, *Animal law: Principles and Frontiers*, published http://bawp.org.au/wp-content/uploads

Mehta, S, M & S, 1990, *Yoga The Iyengar Way*, Dorling Kindersley, London.

Miller, J. 1986 (1982), *Darwin for Beginners*, Writers and Readers Publishing Cooperative in Association with Unwin Paperbacks, London.

Miner, H. Craig. 1976, *The Indian and the Corporation*, Curators of the University of Missouri Press, Columbia (1988 University of Oklahoma Press, Norman, 1989 University of Oklahoma Press).

Oldroyd, D. R . 1980, *Darwinian Impacts: an introduction to the Darwinian Revolution*, The Open University Press, Milton Keynes.

Paramhans Swami Maheshwaranandam 2004 (2002), *The Hidden Power of Humans*, Ibera Verlag/European University Press, Vienna.

Pearson, M. 1998, 'Slaughterhouse', Animals Today, vol 6, no. 2.

Retallack, D. 1973, *The Secret Life of Plants*, DeVorss & Co, California.

Rifkin, J. 1993 (1992), *Beyond Beef: The Rise and Fall of the Cattle Culture*, Plume, Penguin Group, New York.

Rifkin, J. 2013, *The Third Industrial Revolution: How lateral power is transforming energy, the economy, and the world*, Palgrave MacMillan, a division of St. Martin's Press LLC, New York.

Rifkin, J. 2015, *The Zero Cost Marginal Society: The internet of things, the collaborative commons, and the eclipse of capitalism*, Palgrave MacMillan, a division of St. Martin's Press LLC, New York.

Ruse, M. 1999 (1979) *The Darwinian Revolution: Science Red in Tooth and Claw*, University of Chicago, Chicago.

Satyananda Sarasvati, Swami 1985, *Kundalini Tantra*, Satyananda Ashram, Gosford courtesy of Bihar School of Yoga, Bihar.

Singer, P. 1977 (1975), *Animal Liberation*, Granada Publishing Limited, Herts.

Singer, P. 2009, (1975) *Animal Liberation, The definitive classic of the animal movement*, Harper Collins, New York.

Singer, P. 2016, *Ethics in the Real World*, Text Publishing Company, Melbourne.

Spiegel, M. 1988, *The Dreaded Comparison: Human and Animal Slavery*, Mirror Books, United Kingdom.

Wilson, E. O. 1984, *Biophilia*, Harvard University Press, Massachusetts.

Wilson, E. O. 1997 (1996), *In Search of Nature*, Penguin Books, London.

## About the author

The author trained in traditional yoga in 1985 and has since studied different yoga disciplines. Besides being a yoga teacher, she is an award-winning author of women's fiction, a part-time counsellor and member of AMORC (Ancient Mystical Order Rosae Crucis) whose teachings complement those of yoga from a more western perspective.

www.ingramcontent.com/pod-product-compliance
Lightning Source LLC
Chambersburg PA
CBHW041220030426
42336CB00024B/3400